D0529950

Joyce Daly Margie, MD

Co-author of the *Mayo Clinic Renal Diet Cookbook*,
Living with High Blood Pressure, *Living Better*, and
Nutrition in the Cancer Patient, is a nutrition consultant,
formerly at the Mayo Clinic, Rochester, Minnesota

P. J. Palumbo, MD

Consultant, Division of Endocrinology and Metabolism
and Internal Medicine, Mayo Clinic and Mayo Foundation;
Professor of Medicine, Mayo Medical School,
Rochester, Minnesota

The Complete Diabetic Cookbook

JOYCE DALY MARGIE
AND
DR P. J. PALUMBO

Foreword by Professor Harry Keen

Children's Section by
R. Paul Margie

GRAFTON BOOKS

A Division of the Collins Publishing Group

LONDON GLASGOW
TORONTO SYDNEY AUCKLAND

Grafton Books
A Division of the Collins Publishing Group
8 Grafton Street, London W1X 3LA

Published by Grafton Books 1987

British Library Cataloguing in Publication Data
Margie, Joyce Daly
The complete diabetic cookbook.
1. Diabetes—Diet therapy—Recipes
I. Title   II. Palumbo, P. J.
641.5'6314   RC662

ISBN 0-246-12392-3

Printed in Great Britain by
Robert Hartnoll (1985) Ltd, Bodmin, Cornwall

Photoset by Rowland Phototypesetting Ltd,
Bury St Edmunds, Suffolk

NOTE

The recipes in this book are intended for use in
conjunction with the treatment prescribed by the
individual's doctor and in no circumstances should
sufferers discontinue their prescribed treatment.

Contents

Foreword

by Harry Keen

Professor of Human Metabolism,
Director, Unit for Metabolic Medicine,
Guy's Hospital, London

An old aunt of mine summarized her knowledge of dietetics in the simple thesis that 'What don't kill, fattens.' She gave the lie to this simple rule herself for, without effort, she ate indiscriminately, remained lean and was no doubt killed by it all – at the age of 86. She also illustrated the fact (and must herself often have drawn attention to it) that we're all made different. We are also all made very adaptable so that, so long as it is not working under pressure or deprived of the essential nutrient building blocks, the body can work chemical miracles, turning fish to flesh and wine to water. We *could* all live on a comparatively simple daily cocktail of carbohydrate, protein, fat, minerals, vitamins and trace elements which would taste like melted, meat-flavoured ice-cream and give us everything we needed except one thing, enjoyment.

Now we doctors have been telling you patients about diet and diabetes, sometimes through the agency of dietitians, for decades. One problem is that we haven't been telling you the same thing all the time. Not too long ago we were telling you to cut back on the starchy carbohydrates, to cut out sugary carbohydrates, to cut down on all carbohydrates. (Fibre had not been born, but we had roughage.) If you were hungry we told you to fill up on eggs, cheese, butter and cream. Now we advise you to restrict these dairy fat foods and suggest that the bulk of your food energy should come from carbohydrates. Bulk is the right word because carbohydrate with its natural fibre is bulky stuff, heavy to haul home from the supermarket, hard to pack enough into the stomach and heavy in its demands upon the excretory function of the bowel. Diabetics shouldn't feel different in all this. Just the same sort of dietary advice is being given to the population at large. The purpose is to try to reduce the chance of developing arterial disease, coronaries, strokes and gangrene, the main causes of disability and premature death in diabetics and non-diabetics alike.

Food is one of the pleasures of life. We all respond well to its looks, smells and tastes, to the company round the table, to the community it brings, to the memories of home and holidays. We react badly to being deprived of food, to restrictions in choice and in quantity, to loss of the familiar and to being presented with the unaccustomed. We resent the intrusion of the expert into our dietary choices, the medicalization of our meals. But we accept – perhaps with reservations – the seeming rationality of what we are told and seek to maintain our health without losing our *joie de vivre* in the process.

There is only one way through this maze of instinctive drives, learned habits, cultural pressures, economic constraints and fear of disease, and that is understanding. With enough knowledge, the diabetic can have an almost unlimited choice of food. Nothing is forbidden, all is possible, if we can watch our step. That is the purpose of the many books about diet and diabetes and they achieve it with varying measures of success. This book explains not only the way with foods but also how the body handles them and where the diabetic state may interfere. An expert committee of the World Health Organization said that, by acquiring adequate knowledge, every diabetic should become his or her own doctor; the diabetic should become a dietitian too and working through this book will help in that aim.

'Moderation in all things' my old aunt also used to say and certainly that is true in dietary advice for diabetics. It is important to resist the 'over-the-top' approach to diet. The wild consumption of bran and beans will soon pall and diabetics, rejecting it, will find themselves rudderless, disheartened and confused. Fibre is indeed a useful component of diet – we all get some anyway and would probably do well to take a little more. At the very least it will help the bowels. While diabetes is not something to be celebrated it is far from being a disaster, medically, socially or nutritionally. Enjoyment of food is important to the enjoyment of life, and all diabetics, along with everyone else, have the right to enjoy their food. This book will enable them to do so to the full.

Acknowledgements

All nutrient analysis was done at The Ohio State University. Information on their continually updated data base is available from:

> Dianne Clapp, MS, RD
> Department of Dietetics
> Ohio State University Hospital
> 410 West 10th Avenue
> Columbus, Ohio 43210

Jill Metcalfe, who has had extensive experience with diabetics and who is now working for the British Diabetic Association, reviewed the dietary aspects of the manuscript and made suggestions for the British edition. She revised the chapter on planning meals in the British edition and checked and, where necessary, recalculated the nutrient analyses.

Peggy Thielen Schreck, MS, RD, Consultant Nutritionist, Summit, New Jersey, was responsible for coding the recipes for nutritional analysis.

The dietitians at the Mayo Clinic, Saint Marys Hospital and Rochester Methodist Hospital in Rochester, Minnesota, contributed suggestions, guidance and recipes. Virginia Anderson, RD, was particularly helpful.

All recipes were home-tested by our patients, whose ideas and suggestions are greatly appreciated. The recipes in the children's section of the book were also tested by Andrew Margie and Barbara Fleissner.

Preface

Diabetes is not a short-term illness but a chronic disease requiring a lifetime of careful control if serious complications are to be avoided. Whether he or she is taking a drug or not, every diabetic must constantly control the intake of certain nutrients. The purpose of this book is to explain and simplify, for diabetics and their families, the problem of diabetes and how the diet treatment plan can be translated into recipes and cookery.

Until recently, the carbohydrate content of the diabetic's diet was very restricted, and these calories were made up by increasing the fat and protein content. Sugar was strictly forbidden and the use of artificial sweeteners was encouraged. No attention was paid to the cholesterol and fibre content of such diets.

Today, the diabetic patient is instructed to follow a diet that is *low* in fat and cholesterol and *high* in fibre and complex carbohydrates. In addition the diabetic is now permitted limited amounts of sugar.

All these new findings have been taken into consideration in our selection of recipes, which are a balance between simple and more sophisticated fare. They have been chosen on the basis of the *whole family* enjoying the *same* meals rather than cooking special, separate and usually uninteresting dishes for the diabetic member of the family.

Diabetes in children is a special problem. Nutritional therapy in children is particularly difficult because of the child's reluctance to follow the necessary diet restrictions, especially if the diet means that he or she cannot eat the foods that other children enjoy. Therefore we have included a chapter specifically addressed to the medical and nutritional problems of the diabetic child and containing easy-to-follow recipes for dishes favoured by children. This section was written and tested by the teenage son of one of the authors.

We hope that our book will be enjoyed by and helpful to diabetics and their families.

JDM and PJP

PART ONE

Diabetes: the medical problem and its treatment

1. Background Information on Diabetes

The condition called diabetes mellitus is caused by the body's inability to produce enough insulin (some diabetics cannot produce any at all), *or* by the inability of the cells to use the insulin that is produced, *or* by a combination of both. Normally, insulin is produced in the pancreas. The cells that manufacture and release the insulin are the beta cells and are grouped in specific areas of the pancreas called islets. Often the term 'islet cell' is used to refer to the beta cell, but this is not a good term as islets contain cells other than beta cells.

Insulin affects the storage and metabolism of sugar, fat and protein in the body. If it is absent the breakdown of fat is affected and large quantities of molecules called ketoacids are produced. This disturbs the acid balance in the body and can become life-threatening.

Whether the failure to produce insulin is total or partial, the blood sugar level may rise enough to cause increased thirst and frequent urination; the accumulation of ketoacids usually occurs only when the body is not producing any insulin at all.

Protein breakdown can occur with both types of diabetes mellitus. It leads to loss of muscle mass and bone mass.

Choice of treatment depends on the kind of diabetes the patient has – e.g. insulin completely absent, only decreased in amount or present but used inadequately. When there is complete failure of insulin production, insulin injections and special attention to calorie intake, timing of meals and exercise are important to control blood sugar and ketoacid production. If there is only a decrease in insulin production, or an inability to use insulin, diet control alone *may* be enough. However, if diet control alone is not enough, oral medication or insulin may be necessary. Oral medication is not suitable for the diabetic who produces no insulin at all.

Being overweight increases the amount of insulin needed, and there is some evidence that body cells may actually resist the action of insulin in overweight people. So, weight control is an important part of diabetes treatment.

Who Gets Diabetes?
Several forms of diabetes – called secondary diabetes mellitus – result from other diseases. These include inflammation of the pancreas (pancreatitis), glandular (endocrine) disturbances (endrocrine diseases) such as Cushing's disease or excess production of cortisone-like substances, an excess production of growth hormone (acromegaly) which opposes the effects of insulin, and excess production of epinephrine-like substances (pheochromocytoma) which also oppose the effects of insulin.

Heredity plays a part in primary diabetes mellitus and seems to be an important factor in the development of the non-insulin-dependent form in which the body does produce some insulin. Diabetes may be present in parents, children and the siblings of people with non-insulin-dependent diabetes. If one identical twin has non-insulin-dependent diabetes the condition will almost certainly develop in the other.

Other influences – such as diet, viral infections or something yet to be identified – may play a role in the development of insulin-dependent diabetes, the form in which the body produces no insulin.

The Role of Diet
Diet has long been recognized as a key component in the care of diabetics and there has been much controversy about the best diet for them. But there is now agreement on general

underlying principles. Most authorities agree that the goals of diet therapy are the following: (1) to help adjust for metabolic abnormalities, (2) to help prevent vascular complications in blood circulation and (3) to provide safe flexibility to allow for individual lifestyles and differences in tastes and economic resources.

We now know that when insulin is present a relatively high intake of carbohydrates actually improves blood sugar control by enhancing sensitivity to insulin. Diets high in carbohydrates help both insulin-dependent and non-insulin-dependent diabetics. Another effect of increasing carbohydrate content has been the decrease in calories from fat and protein. The metabolism of excessive fat and protein may contribute to cardiovascular disease, the main cause of death among diabetics.

Every diabetic has individual nutritional needs that should be determined by the doctor and dietitian. Meals should be consistent from day to day in content, number and timing. This is important whatever the type of diabetes. So each diabetic should spend some time with a dietitian who can help work out an appropriate diet plan. Your doctor can refer you to a dietitian specializing in diets for diabetics.

Exercise
Regular exercise should be a routine part of the diabetic's life but sporadic exercise has little value. Regular exercise can be beneficial in several ways: it may reduce resistance to insulin; it may help control weight; it may reduce the factors that could lead to heart disease. Exercise enhances work capacity and promotes good muscle conditioning, physical fitness and a feeling of well-being.

Because exercise tends to lower blood sugar concentration, insulin-dependent diabetics may need to adjust their insulin dosage to prevent hypoglycaemia. Chapter 5 presents a more detailed discussion of exercise.

The Patient's Role in Managing Diabetes

Patients must take part wholeheartedly in managing their diabetes. It is not enough just to show up for doctors' appointments and blindly follow the regimen. The doctor and the dietitian must stay in touch with the patient. Diabetes is a lifelong disorder and will not go away, so the diabetic's best chance of leading a 'normal life' is to make sure that the prescribed diet, exercise and medication suit his or her way of life as far as possible.

This means that a diabetic must be absolutely truthful with the other members of the team. Tell your dietitian exactly what you eat and don't eat, when you like to eat, and whether or not you can obtain the foods suggested at the time suggested.

Unless the patient is quite young it will probably not be possible to change eating patterns drastically. The dietitian is well equipped by education and training to help work out a programme suiting an individual's lifestyle.

The nurses and doctors working with you cannot read your mind. If you have fears, problems or questions, discuss them, even if you consider them 'silly'. You are probably not the first or the last person to ask the same things. No question relating to a person's health is 'silly'.

The better informed the patient and the family are, and the better prepared to meet unexpected or expected situations, the more successful will be the control of the disease.

The Future

In the past few years there has been much discussion about the classification of diabetes into its insulin-dependent and non-insulin-dependent forms. Discussion and research have centred on the relationship of these forms to hereditary factors, complications and long-term outcome. The hope has been that, through accurate classification, we may predict the course of the disease and provide more specific treatment.

Unfortunately, the present classification is not precise enough for this.

Diabetes probably represents not two but ten or more different types of disorder in which high blood sugar levels are found. As we become able to define each specific type, the physician will be able to predict the course and outcome and prescribe specific treatment that may prevent complications.

It is also hoped that physicians will eventually be able to identify those in whom diabetes *will* develop and to take steps to prevent it. At present the early identification of latent or 'hidden' diabetes is of little use because not much help can be offered other than weight reduction for the obese. Medical science has no definitive treatment programme by which early diagnosis can halt the development of the symptoms or complications of diabetes.

The most exciting future prospect is the possibility of using 'genetic engineering', either to get insulin production started again in the case of the damaged beta cells or to provide new cells that will produce insulin.

Whatever the future of diabetes treatment – with insulin, oral agents, artificial devices, transplantation or genetic engineering – diet remains the mainstay of all treatments and this is particularly important for those whose diabetes can be controlled by calorie restriction, weight reduction and regular exercise.

2. Insulin-dependent Diabetes Mellitus

Insulin-dependent diabetes mellitus is a disorder in which there is complete absence of insulin production by the beta cells of the pancreas. Some research indicates that this happens in people genetically prone to a viral infection that leads to destruction of the beta cells. But this hypothesis has not been proved, and at present there is no way to identify people who are most susceptible to such infections.

Diabetes mellitus is usually first recognized when the patient experiences constant increased urination and increased thirst. The increase includes greater frequency of urination as well as a greater quantity of urine each time. This loss of water from the body causes the thirst, and increased drinking to quench the thirst further increases urination. With the increased urination there is loss of sugar leading to loss of calories and, therefore, usually a loss of weight, even when the appetite is hearty and food intake adequate.

If these symptoms are ignored or go unrecognized the water loss becomes drastic and there is also a loss of important chemicals and a growing acidity in the blood. If the disease is still not recognized the patient steadily weakens, becomes lethargic and may lapse into coma and die.

A patient may think the symptoms reflect a viral infection such as flu, and will pass with time. Therefore persistent symptoms and worsening of the patient's condition signal that medical attention is needed. If members of the family are known diabetics the investigation of such symptoms is urgent.

A seasonal variation in the development of insulin-dependent diabetes, particularly in children, is more likely to occur during autumn and winter which increases the danger of its being confused with flu. The patient may indeed have flu also, and this can mask the underlying diabetes. Usually flu is an illness of the upper respiratory tract, and gastro-intestinal symptoms should alert one to the possibility of diabetes as nausea and vomiting may be caused by excess production of ketoacids.

Heredity may play a role in the development of insulin-dependent diabetes mellitus. Research has shown an increased frequency of diabetes in the siblings of diabetics and in identical twins. Also, some genetic markers have been identified, such as human leukocyte antigens, which identify individuals who may be more prone to diabetes. Whether these individuals are more susceptible to infections which lead to islet cell destruction is not yet clear.

How Is Diabetes Diagnosed?
Diagnosis of diabetes is made by measuring the blood glucose (sugar) level. According to the British Diabetic Association (BDA), a random venous plasma value of 11 mmol/L or more or a fasting value of 8 mmol/L or more indicates diabetes. In insulin-dependent patients, there is usually little doubt about the diagnosis because the blood glucose level will be dramatically high, usually more than 11 mmol/L, and there will be sugar in the urine. In fact a urine test is almost as good as a blood test for diagnosing the disease. A patient with the symptoms described above and sugar present in the urine will probably have a blood sugar level greater than 11 mmol/L. Normal people have no sugar in the urine.

To detect insulin-dependent diabetes special testing is not necessary. Such patients are more likely to have the symptoms, with abnormal thirst and urination and greatly increased blood sugar levels. They also have the most reliable sign of diabetes: fasting hyperglycaemia (blood sugar level is

8 mmol/L or more after an overnight fast). Detecting fasting hyperglycaemia requires only one blood test done at least 12 hours after the last meal the night before. The test should be done on two separate days to be sure that the first report is not mistaken.

A glucose tolerance test is not necessary. In this test a glucose load or meal is given and the blood sugar level then measured repeatedly over a 3- to 5-hour period. This is an artificial test of how the body handles blood sugar, and there are instances in which the test has given an abnormal result though the patient never developed full-blown diabetes. The best test remains the measurement of blood sugar after a 12-hour overnight fast.

With no insulin production and high blood sugar levels, fat breakdown occurs at an increased rate in the insulin-dependent diabetic, leading to the production of ketoacids (ketoacidosis) exceeding the body's ability to use them. The ketoacids are therefore flushed out in the urine, leading to further water loss.

These substances can be measured in the urine, and the presence of sugar and ketoacids in the urine is strong evidence that the patient has a marked increase in the blood sugar level. When ketoacidosis is present along with high blood sugar levels, regardless of the time of day, the two fasting blood sugar tests are unnecessary for diagnosis.

Treatment
The immediate aim of treatment is to restore the blood sugar level to normal or near normal. The long-term goal is to prevent the acute and chronic complications of diabetes.

Rapid changes in blood sugar levels may be harmful to various organs. The treatment programme must prevent a blood sugar level above 11 mmol/L for anything more than 15 to 30 minutes. Current preference is to maintain the level between 4–7 mmol/L before meals and at not more than 8.5 mmol/L after meals.

One approach to the control of blood sugar level uses 'self blood glucose monitoring'. This is done by the patient, who pricks a finger to obtain a drop of capillary blood, places the blood on a strip of paper and compares the colour change with a standard scale. The doctor instructs the patient on how to adjust insulin dosage on the basis of these tests.

Testing urine for sugar is done less frequently, but tests for ketoacids in urine are used in conjunction with self blood glucose monitoring to determine whether a particular blood sugar level is accompanied by ketoacid production, in which case an aggressive treatment programme may be needed to avert disaster.

Another measure of control is the sugar content of haemoglobin in the blood (glycosylated haemoglobin level). When the blood sugar level increases so does the glycosylated haemoglobin level. This measurement gives an estimate of diabetes control for a longer period than does a single blood sugar test. Currently the test is carried out at intervals of two to three months and provides information about the diabetes control for the previous one to three months. In future it may be possible to measure glycosylated haemoglobin on capillary blood specimens, as is now being done for glucose. The goal of therapy is to keep the glycosylated haemoglobin within the normal range, usually between 4 and 7 per cent depending on the laboratory performing the test.

Dietary Management
Diet control and insulin therapy begin as soon as insulin-dependent diabetes is diagnosed. The diet is based on the patient's weight and caloric need. Most insulin-dependent diabetics are lean, so their diet is tailored to provide the calories needed to maintain ideal weight. If patients are underweight an attempt is made to increase calories and bring their weight up to the ideal for their age, body frames and activities. (See Appendix for weight chart.) An overweight patient gets a calorie-restricted diet to decrease weight and

thereby provide an optimal effect of the insulin therapy.

Frequency and timing of meals are co-ordinated with the insulin therapy. Most insulin-taking patients need a bedtime snack in addition to breakfast, lunch and dinner. Because of the time at which the injected insulin has its maximum effect on the blood sugar, a mid-afternoon meal may also be needed. A mid-morning meal is often necessary because of the use of fast-acting insulin before breakfast. The marked variability in blood sugar levels cannot be entirely explained by the action of the insulin itself, but an additional meal will help to maintain the blood sugar. The absorption of insulin from the site of injection is an important factor in the speed and duration of the insulin effect. This absorption can vary from day to day and according to the site of injection (for example, leg versus abdomen).

The total calorie intake for insulin-dependent diabetics is determined by the ideal weight. For the overweight patient a calorie-restricted diet may be prescribed. The calorie intake needs to be distributed throughout the day in amounts matching the times of the insulin effect and must provide a mixture of carbohydrate with protein or fat or both at each meal. For the controlled individual close to ideal weight, continued weight loss or unusual weight gain indicate a visit to the doctor or dietitian to revise the diet.

What type of carbohydrate should be used is discussed in later chapters, but in general there is a tendency to provide much of it in complex forms with fibre to avoid too rapid absorption and quick upswings in blood sugar level. Protein and fat in the diet are also discussed later. Mixed meals, comprising carbohydrates, fats and protein, slow down the absorption of carbohydrate and so allow smoother control of the blood sugar level.

Management with Insulin
The insulin needed by insulin-dependent diabetics comes in several varieties. Some preparations contain insulin from

animals such as cows or pigs; some are mixtures of both. Synthesized human insulin is now available and is usually recommended for new insulin-dependent diabetics, but it is not necessary to change from your current insulin to human insulin.

Insulin preparations can also be classed in terms of their duration of action. Currently available preparations are quick-acting, intermediate-acting and long-acting. Quick-acting insulin has an effect for 3 to 6 hours, intermediate-acting insulin for 18 to 24 hours and long-acting insulin for 24 to 36 hours. Some others, such as semilente insulin, act for 6 to 12 hours.

Quick-acting, or standard, insulin comes as a clear solution. The intermediate- and long-acting insulins are in suspension. Insulins in suspension must be shaken before use.

Insulin-dependent patients will often need two injections per day, about two-thirds of the insulin being taken before breakfast and a third before the evening meal – but exact proportions are determined by the doctor, as they vary with the individual. Some patients may need the same amount of insulin before breakfast and the evening meal, and may also need to combine quick-acting and intermediate-acting insulins in the same syringe each time. Such information is given by the doctor when deciding the dosage for best control.

In more intensified treatments a patient may need a quick-acting insulin dose before each meal and a long-acting dose in the evening or before breakfast. The daily dosages of quick-acting and long-acting insulin are determined by self blood glucose monitoring, which imitates the natural monitoring of sugar level by the beta cell of the pancreas, which then responds by producing insulin to control the blood sugar.

Insulin infusion pumps now used by some patients provide a continuous infusion of insulin but require close medical supervision for the adjustment of doses between and at meal-times.

There are special insulin injector devices that can be helpful to patients with impaired vision, but none of these injector devices has any advantage over the insulin injection programme or insulin pump.

Oral hypoglycaemic agents are not appropriate treatment for insulin-dependent diabetics, as they depend on insulin production by the patient's pancreas.

Complications in Insulin Treatment
The most common complication in insulin treatment is low blood sugar (hypoglycaemia), usually called 'insulin reaction' or 'hypo'. The usual symptoms are sweating, irritability, palpitations, blurred vision, hunger and headaches.

Hypoglycaemia may result from taking too much insulin, insufficient food, delayed meals or over-exercise. It must be treated promptly by taking a simple carbohydrate, such as sugar in water or orange juice, a special sugar preparation that can be swallowed easily or any item from the list below.

Fluid	*Amount to be taken*
Lucozade, or similar glucose drink	50 ml/2 fl oz
Grape juice (natural bottled)	50 ml/2 fl oz
Fruit juices (natural unsweetened), 1 wine glass	100 ml/4 fl oz
Coke or Pepsi, 1 wine glass	100 ml/4 fl oz
Lemonade, or similar carbonated drink	150 ml/5 fl oz
Milk, 1 cup	200 ml/7 fl oz
Soup (thickened creamed, e.g. chicken), 1 cup	200 ml/7 fl oz
Soup (tomato, tinned), ½ cup	100 ml/4 fl oz

Low-calorie diet drinks or diet foods will not correct hypoglycaemia. See your doctor regarding the proper treatment. It is important to learn to recognize hypoglycaemia and treat it promptly.

When hypoglycaemia is more severe – producing confusion or inability to respond – it may be necessary to inject sugar intravenously or administer the hormone glucagon which stimulates the production of sugar in the body.

The treatment of hypoglycaemia should never be delayed and prompt recognition and treatment of the severe condition by relatives or friends are vital. If it is not treated promptly the patient could have serious complications.

Another complication of insulin treatment is the development of antibodies to the insulin. These are more likely to develop when animal insulin, particularly bovine, is used. High antibody levels stop the insulin from affecting the blood sugar level. Your doctor can advise you about treatment for high antibody levels, but with present-day highly purified insulin preparations, particularly the human insulin ones, excess antibodies should not occur, or only rarely.

Skin reaction to injected insulin is another possible complication. Most skin reactions appear in the area of the injection and occur within some six weeks of the start of insulin therapy. The reactions usually clear spontaneously and need no specific treatment. The occasional injection of Benadryl along with insulin may help to reduce localized skin reaction, but the mere continuation of insulin injections may reduce skin reaction in time.

Another skin reaction to injected insulin is the loss of subcutaneous fat or the excess accumulation of it. These changes usually show up in the area of injection. The build-up of fat is more likely in men, the loss more likely in women. Again, with today's highly purified insulin preparations, particularly the human insulin ones, such reactions should become uncommon.

A few patients may develop insulin allergy. It can manifest itself through generalized hives, swelling of the lips or difficult breathing. Patients who have had an allergy or eczema in infancy or childhood may be susceptible to insulin allergy, while starting and stopping insulin may produce an allergic response in certain individuals. If you suspect such a reaction you should see your doctor.

Effects of Other Medications

Diabetics may be taking treatment for other conditions and some drugs, such as cortisone, affect the action of insulin. The insulin dosage may need adjusting when such medication is used.

When the patient is on such medications as the beta-adrenergic blocking agents which are often used in heart disease, the insulin reaction may not be recognized or the body may produce insufficient sugar to overcome the reaction.

Your doctor can best advise you about interaction between other medications and your insulin programme.

Pregnancy in the Diabetic

An insulin-dependent diabetic who is pregnant must have sufficient insulin and nutrition to prevent ketoacidosis, a condition especially hazardous to the growing foetus. It is also essential that blood sugar levels be kept normal or near-normal.

Diabetes control should be rigorous from the very start of pregnancy to prevent malformations of the organ systems that develop in the foetus in the first 12 weeks. Good control later in the pregnancy promotes healthy growth of the foetus and a healthy child at birth. High blood sugar levels in the mother make the beta cells of the foetus over-sensitive to blood sugar levels, a condition associated with hypoglycaemia in the newborn which can cause brain damage and lead to death. The baby of a diabetic mother must be monitored carefully for developing hypoglycaemia.

Keeping the blood sugar level nearly normal in the diabetic

mother will also prevent an excess of fluid and fat in the baby that can make delivery difficult, and control of the mother's diabetes also prevents immaturity of the foetus's organ systems. A major cause of death of infants born to diabetic mothers is lung problems, and good control of the mother's diabetes can reduce this risk.

There is a form of diabetes that occurs only during pregnancy: gestational diabetes, which may increase the risk of such pregnancy complications as toxaemia, high blood pressure and excess amniotic fluid (hydramnios) and can result in a large baby which is difficult to deliver and prone to birth injury. It may also heighten the risk of congenital malformation, birth defects and lung disease in the newborn. A woman with gestational diabetes during pregnancy has a fairly high chance of developing diabetes later in life.

The treatment for gestational diabetes is a nutritious diet with calories adequate for growth of the foetus and prevention of ketosis. Insulin treatment may be necessary if the fasting blood sugar level is more than 5.5 mmol/L and if the sugar level two hours after a meal is more than 7 mmol/L.

Motoring and the Diabetic
Hypoglycaemia (insulin reaction) or a low blood sugar level poses a special hazard to the diabetic motorist. Food should be available in the car and meals should not be skipped during a driving trip. At the slightest suspicion of an insulin reaction coming on, food should be taken.

Fortunately, insulin reactions are not a major problem for most diabetics on insulin, but they *can* be. The diabetic driver needs to be aware of this potential problem when he or she gets behind the wheel of a car. The British Diabetic Association recommends the following:

Tell your insurance company that you are diabetic.

State on the application for a licence that you are diabetic.

Always carry carbohydrate in the car.

Never drink and drive.

Eat your usual carbohydrate allowance less than two hours before setting off.

At the first symptoms of a 'hypo', STOP driving and remove the ignition key. Take carbohydrate immediately. In order to make it clear that you are no longer in charge of the car, you would be well advised to get out of the car until the symptoms have disappeared. This should refute any suggestion that you are in charge of a car whilst under the influence of drugs.

The British Diabetic Association further cautions that you should not drive if:

You are being stabilized on insulin – until stabilization is complete.

You have difficulty in recognizing early symptoms of a 'hypo', which may affect your judgement and lead to aggressive behaviour, poor muscle control, and even sudden unconsciousness.

You have any problems with your eyesight that cannot be corrected by glasses or have numbness or weakness in your limbs due to diabetic nerve disease.

Infections
A high blood sugar level – i.e. above 16.5 mmol/L – impairs the activity of the white blood cells and other defence mechanisms that fight infection in the body. Thus when diabetes is poorly regulated infections of the skin, urinary tract, vagina and penis are more likely to develop. Infections of the vagina and penis are usually fungal infections. Infections of the skin and urinary tract are usually caused by bacteria. Drugs used for treating both kinds of infection are more effective when the blood sugar is controlled.

Diabetic Ketoacidosis
The major acute complication of insulin-dependent diabetes is diabetic ketoacidosis, the condition resulting from too little insulin in the body because of inadequate dosage. First a high

blood sugar level develops, then the high blood sugar and the inability to use it through lack of insulin trigger excess production of ketoacids as products of fat breakdown. Next come disturbances in water metabolism, electrolytes and acid content of the blood. When ketoacidosis develops there is increased thirst, frequent urination, nausea, vomiting, increased breathing or overbreathing and a state of weakness, fatigue and lethargy. The symptoms usually develop in a few days, and if they go unrecognized the patient may lapse into coma and die. The condition calls for hospitalization and prompt intravenous treatment with fluids and insulin.

These days deaths from ketoacidosis are few because it is quickly recognized – by the patient, by relatives and by doctors. The doctor should be contacted immediately if the condition is suspected.

Long-term Complications
Complications can occur in any diabetic but are more likely when diabetes is poorly controlled.

In one form, microangiopathy (disease of small blood vessels), the small vessels of the eye become damaged and any new vessels that form are of poor quality. They cause bleeding within the chamber of the eye which leads to blindness. The bleeding may lead to increased pressure, or glaucoma, and the eye may have to be removed. Blood vessel changes related to diabetes may be controlled by their early recognition and early treatment with laser photocoagulation, so frequent eye examinations are important.

The small blood vessels of the kidney, too, may be affected. This leads to loss of protein through the urine and eventually to kidney failure, which may make it necessary for the patient to undergo dialysis regularly. Even a kidney transplant may become necessary. Diet changes may be made when a patient has kidney failure. Carbohydrate is increased, protein reduced and salt is restricted.

Damage to the nerves in the legs may occur with diabetes,

and seems to be related to a loss of the covering of the nerves. Sometimes the blood supply to the nerves is impaired, leading to changes in their function. When the nerves are affected, pain may be felt in the feet and legs and the legs may become weak. There may be damage to the nerves controlling the eye muscles. When this happens – rarely – pain and weakness may affect the eye.

Fortunately the symptoms caused by these changes to the nerves will gradually go away. No specific treatment is necessary, though pain-killing drugs or tranquillizers may occasionally be necessary to control the more severe symptoms.

Damage to the nerves to the feet may cause a loss of sensation and an unawareness of any injury to the feet. This can lead to ulceration, infection and, ultimately, to loss of the foot or leg. Thus it is very important to inspect the feet frequently and to be certain that all footwear fits properly, with no rubbing that might cause ulceration. Shoes should also be checked for foreign bodies before being put on. Foot care is important in the treatment of diabetes.

There can be damage to the nerves controlling the heart rate or those controlling the blood vessels. When these nerves are damaged, the heart rate will increase and the blood pressure may drop when the patient stands up, perhaps causing dizziness. In diabetic men there may be damage to the nerve controlling penile erections, causing impotence.

Another major complication of diabetes is macroangiopathy, disease of the large blood vessels. This can involve the arteries to the heart, the legs and the brain. Arteriosclerosis (hardening of the arteries) develops. The arteries become narrower, which impairs circulation and reduces the amount of blood reaching the organ systems. The result can be heart attack, gangrene or stroke. Special diet modifications may be necessary for patients with such a condition.

Other Risk Factors
In treating diabetes it is important to correct other factors that increase the risk of blood vessel disease. Diabetics should not smoke. High blood pressure should be corrected by control of the salt intake and appropriate medication. High blood cholesterol or triglyceride level or both should also be corrected, though high triglyceride level may result from poor regulation of the diabetes. If cholesterol and triglyceride levels remain high despite good control of the diabetes specific treatment may be needed. Overweight patients need to reduce body weight, and this alone may correct high blood pressure and high blood cholesterol and triglyceride levels.

Possible Future Treatment
The search goes on for more effective treatment – to restore beta cell function or to mimic it more closely.

Pancreas transplants have had limited success and are still under investigation. Beta cells have been isolated from the pancreas but attempts at implanting them in humans have not succeeded.

A computer program being developed will mimic the activity of the beta cell in recognizing the blood sugar level and responding with an appropriate amount of insulin. The program will be housed in a small device implanted in the body and will act as an artificial beta cell.

Another idea, based on genetic engineering, is to reprogram defective beta cells to produce insulin again, or to program other cells in the body to do the work of beta cells. The production of insulin in bacteria makes this form of treatment more of a reality than might be anticipated.

Relationship Between Doctor and Diabetic Patient
It is important to have a doctor – preferably one specializing in diabetes – readily available and accessible, especially when the patient is having difficulties or is ill. The diabetic must also be able to discuss freely with the doctor any problems that arise.

An open and honest relationship with the doctor is important in helping the diabetic cope with the disease and the treatment. If you have difficulty finding such a doctor, contact the British Diabetic Association for a list of diabetes specialists in your area.

3. Non-insulin-dependent Diabetes Mellitus

Non-insulin-dependent diabetes mellitus is the condition in which the patient's body produces insulin but not enough to control the blood sugar level. This can indicate defective production of insulin or resistance by the body's cells to the action of insulin.

Diabetics of this type are less likely to have ketoacidosis. More than half the patients with non-insulin-dependent diabetes are overweight, and diet control alone will treat their condition. Another 20 to 30 per cent will require insulin treatment to control blood sugar level and some 10 to 20 per cent will have to take certain drugs by mouth.

Goals of Treatment

The immediate goal of treatment is to achieve normal or near normal blood sugar levels. The long-term aim is to prevent the acute and chronic complications of diabetes. How to translate the immediate goal of therapy into blood sugar levels is described in Chapter 2. Current practice is to maintain blood sugar value between 4 and 7 mmol/L before meals and at no more than 8.5 mmol/L after meals. The glyco-sylated haemoglobin level, which provides an integrated measure of diabetes control over some two to three months, should be within the normal range.

Dietary Management

Dietary principles for the non-insulin-dependent patient recommended by the British Diabetic Association are: 50 per

cent or more of the calorie intake should be from carbohydrates, 15 per cent from protein, and around 30–35 per cent
from fat. Complex carbohydrates with integral fibre should
provide a large part of the carbohydrate intake.

For overweight diabetics a reduced calorie diet (rarely less
than 800 calories) will provide a balanced intake and reduce
weight. Calorie intake for overweight diabetics as for the lean,
non-insulin-dependent diabetic is based on their diet history.
Between-meal snacks should not be necessary unless insulin
therapy is used. A three-meal-per-day plan with the correct
calorie or carbohydrate distribution should suffice unless the
patient prefers several lighter meals.

Insulin Management
Insulin is the best treatment for diabetes when diet control
alone does not keep the blood sugar level down. Insulin
action, insulin preparations and other aspects of insulin treatment are described in Chapter 2.

Most non-insulin-dependent diabetics will require only
one insulin injection per day, though occasionally more than
one may be necessary.

The complications of insulin treatment discussed in Chapter 2 affect the non-insulin-dependent diabetic on insulin as
much as the insulin-dependent patient. Hypoglycaemic reactions are not well tolerated by older patients and may affect
the mental functions or mimic a stroke.

Oral Medication
For the non-insulin-dependent patient whose blood sugar level
does not respond to diet control alone, an oral hypoglycaemic
agent can be taken by mouth. Two kinds of such oral agents
are now available: the sulfonylurea drugs and the biguanide
drugs. Sulfonylurea drugs boost the production of insulin by
the beta cell and make the body more receptive to the insulin.
Biguanides reduce sugar absorption and production and
may affect the use of sugar by the cells. Sulfonylureas and

biguanides can be combined to correct high blood sugar levels.

Both types of oral drugs have a high failure rate. Patients become resistant to their effects and need to change to insulin treatment. One reason for the failure of these drugs is thought to be poor adherence to the diet, and it is important that diabetics taking this type of drug stick to the prescribed diet faithfully. Other reasons these agents fail to maintain long-term control of blood sugar level may relate to a loss of effect on insulin production or on the response of body cells.

Hypoglycaemic reactions may occur in non-insulin-dependent patients who take a sulfonylurea drug. Recognition and treatment of such reactions is discussed in Chapter 2 but if they occur the patient should see a doctor.

Exercise
Regular exercise is important in treating non-insulin-dependent diabetes. Exercise plus an appropriate diet may be enough to control the blood sugar level. Exercise ensures better use of sugar in the body, decreases insulin need and promotes good body tone, general fitness and better circulation to the organ systems.

For an older non-insulin-dependent patient walking two to four miles a day is excellent exercise, if he or she is not overweight. For the overweight patient exercises affecting the large joints may damage them. For such patients swimming and physical fitness programmes may be necessary. For information on exercise and its influence on calorie expenditure see Chapter 5.

Effects of Other Medications
Patients with non-insulin-dependent diabetes are often older and so more likely to be under treatment for other conditions. Such patients must identify all the drugs they are taking and discuss them with their doctor. This helps doctors to spot potential interactions that may cause problems. Possible interactions of other medications with insulin treatment are discussed in Chapter 2.

Travel

For the diabetic being treated by diet alone no special precautions are necessary while travelling other than to keep to the diet and, similarly, the non-insulin-dependent diabetic taking an oral hypoglycaemic agent need only continue taking the drug in line with the suggestions on special situations in Chapter 9.

Oral treatment should pose no particular problem for motoring patients, but sulfonylureas may cause hypoglycaemic reactions so these patients should follow the precautions outlined in Chapter 2 for patients on insulin.

The travel guidelines in Chapter 2 for insulin-dependent patients are appropriate also for the non-insulin-dependent diabetics taking insulin.

Illness

When a diabetic patient, treated by diet alone, becomes ill, testing urine for sugar and ketoacids is necessary, and during an acute illness the patient may need insulin treatment. Similarly, insulin may be necessary during serious illness for a diabetic on an oral agent, and the blood and urine sugar levels and the urine ketoacid level should be checked.

The guidelines in Chapter 9 for insulin-dependent patients also apply to non-insulin-dependent patients on insulin who become ill.

Infection

High blood sugar can impair the body's defences against infection. Comments in Chapter 2 are appropriate also for non-insulin-dependent diabetics.

Coma

Diabetic ketoacidosis is unusual among non-insulin-dependent patients but when it does occur, recognition and management are the same as for insulin-dependent patients (Chapter 2).

More likely for non-insulin-dependent diabetics whose condition is poorly regulated is hyperosmolar nonketotic coma, a complication occurring when enough insulin circulates to prevent the breakdown of body fat into ketoacids but not enough to control the blood sugar level. With dehydration present, as in illness with fever, the blood sugar level may increase to 55 mmol/L or higher. This, combined with the dehydration, leads to lethargy and coma which, if not corrected, may cause the patient to die. The condition is treated by giving the patient water – by mouth if possible, or special fluids intravenously if the patient cannot drink – while small doses of insulin will help to correct the blood sugar level and the patient should recover. At any suspicion that this condition is developing a doctor should be consulted at once.

Long-term Complications

For the non-insulin-dependent diabetic, the most frequent long-term complication is the development of large blood vessel disease (macroangiopathy) affecting the arteries to the heart, legs and brain. The patient may also sustain nerve damage (neuropathy) as described in Chapter 2. Blood vessel changes in the eye or in the kidney (microangiopathy) are rarer among non-insulin-dependent patients, but when they do occur they follow the same course as in insulin-dependent diabetics. Long-term complications in diabetes are dealt with generally in Chapter 2.

Patient and Doctor

Your doctor should be contacted promptly whenever difficulties arise in controlling the diabetes or when illness occurs. At such times patients not on insulin may need it to control high blood sugar levels and other symptoms. Also important is the ability to discuss with your doctor any problems that may be causing you concern. Good relations with your doctor help you to cope.

5. Exercise

Exercise is important in treating diabetes mellitus of whatever type and whatever the type of treatment. Exercise helps to control the blood sugar level throughout the day and many non-insulin-dependent diabetics who exercise regularly and control their weight find medication no longer necessary.

Yet control of the blood sugar level is not the only benefit from exercise. It also promotes physical well-being, good muscle conditioning and better circulation to the organ systems, improving the quality of life and perhaps prolonging it.

In planning an exercise programme, the factors considered are: age, weight, current physical condition, possible physical impediments, individual interests, the timing of exercise and its effect on blood sugar levels.

Age is significant when choosing exercises. Older people tend to be more sedentary than the young, and tests may be necessary to assess physical condition, ability to perform an exercise, and the possible adverse effect of exercise on the heart. Such testing may not be necessary for young diabetics.

Barring physical handicaps, walking and swimming are good exercises for any age group. More vigorous pursuits like cycling, contact sports or tennis demand good physical fitness, and before fully taking part in such sports the patient's physical condition must be gradually improved. Isometric and other exercises that develop muscle also need prior conditioning and a gradual build-up to the full exercise programme.

All exercise should start with a warm-up period of several

panying growth spurt, insulin needs increase. Poor regulation of insulin-dependent diabetes causes ketoacidosis, especially during the period of rapid growth.

'Why Me?'

The emotional impact of having diabetes is very serious for a growing child or adolescent, and tends to impair the young patient's attention to the details of care. Feelings of isolation, of being different, of being singled out by having diabetes are fertile ground for long-term emotional and behavioural problems. To be reminded daily, by details of diet and medication, that one is diabetic, with constraints on one's freedom, can affect the developing personality of the young patient. Indeed, every diabetic, young or old, asks: 'Why me?'

Even with a strongly supportive family young diabetics feel rejected, unloved, victims of unjust circumstances. Anger is followed by 'acting-out' behaviour detrimental to their health, as if they are testing whether the limits imposed by diabetes are real.

Some young diabetics will refuse to carry out the tests needed to monitor diabetes. Some skip their insulin or gradually reduce the doses. Others refuse to vary the injection sites and continually inject insulin in a small area which soon becomes insensitive. Many cheat on their diets, and others will provide fake test results to appear to conform.

Unfortunately all such behaviour means poor regulation of the illness, and uncontrolled diabetes can lead to ketoacidosis, coma and death.

Some young diabetics paradoxically use their condition to obtain the love and attention they feel they have lost because of it. Feelings of inadequacy, rejection and victimization plague the young diabetic, and only with strong support from parents, other family members, doctor and community can the patient be brought to appreciate the more positive aspects of life.

The rebellious attitudes of normal adolescence are compounded in the young diabetic, who in trying to demonstrate independence may unwittingly do things that have dangerous long-term consequences.

It is important that long-term adolescent patients assume responsibility for their health and take pride in their ability to deal with a serious problem. Many join support groups of other diabetics who are experiencing the same feelings and problems, and find it a great help.

Most young diabetics can handle their disorder, given emotional support, and go on to lead happy and productive adult lives.

School

For most young diabetics there are no limits to school activities other than those related to diet and insulin treatment.

A sympathetic teacher can discreetly arrange mid-morning and mid-afternoon snacks and can also note and report behavioural changes that signal poor regulation of the illness – either high or low blood sugar level. The British Diabetic Association has information available that can be used in schools.

It is important for the young diabetic to take part in all normal school activities, including athletics, which should be encouraged. Some fine athletes are diabetics, proving that the condition need be no bar to success in competitive sports. Attention must be paid to the possibility of hypoglycaemic reactions during exercise, and if school staff are properly briefed, errors in judgement can be contained and treatment given when necessary.

The child who cannot get an appropriate meal at school can bring lunch from home, but it is important for young diabetics to join in the activities of other young people, so efforts should be made to enable them to eat the same meals as the others.

Young diabetics must learn to select appropriate meals, as well as snacks after school and at parties. The aim is to minimize the differences between the diabetic child and other children though, at the same time, making it clear that he or she is responsible for the control of the illness.

Career Counselling

Career counselling should start early to decide which of the young diabetic's skills may most usefully be developed for eventual successful employment. An unskilled diabetic on the job market faces a dismal future.

4. Diabetes Mellitus in Children and Adolescents

Diabetes mellitus in children and young people under 18 may affect physical growth and emotional development. Managing diabetes in these young patients requires co-operation between the patient, the medical team, the parents and members of the community – the school nurse and teachers. But final responsibility remains with the patient, and parents must ensure that the diabetic child knows everything they know about the illness. Even very young patients must know the warning signs and treatment for hypoglycaemia and ketoacidosis and should be encouraged to be responsible for themselves as soon as they can. Most children are quite capable, and many – particularly adolescents – do not want parents hovering about, trying to control all aspects of their lives.

When diabetes develops in a person under 18, it is almost always the insulin-dependent type, and treatment is as described in Chapter 2. Important information is also given in the chapters on exercise, special situations and nutritional therapy.

The young diabetic must understand the importance of blood sugar monitoring, regular exercise and adjustment of insulin dosage.

Good control of the condition is necessary for normal metabolism and health. Before puberty the body is extremely sensitive to insulin, and usually only very small doses will maintain normal or nearly normal blood sugar levels and protein and fat metabolism. During puberty and the accom-

minutes and end with an equal cooling-down period to allow favourable transitions between non-active and active states.

Physical Condition

Weight is an important factor in planning an exercise programme. For overweight individuals such exercises as walking may cause or aggravate problems with the knee and foot joints, and isometric or body-building exercises or swimming are probably more appropriate.

The heart, eyes and feet are also important to consider when planning an exercise programme. Severe heart disease, with the inability to move without pain or shortness of breath, limits drastically the amount and type of exercise that can be undertaken, while arthritis or other joint conditions make certain kinds of exercise obviously undesirable. The wrong exercise may aggravate arthritis. A diabetic with severe blood vessel disease of the eye must avoid vigorous exercise to prevent bleeding into the eye.

The diabetic who has foot ulcers, has had a stroke or has damage to the peripheral nerves (neuropathy) should engage in exercises that do not produce pressure on body areas prone to ulceration. Swimming or programmes of body-building and muscle conditioning are suitable for patients with foot problems or neuropathy.

Timing of Exercise

Exercise generally lowers the blood sugar level, but the drop varies in different people because they exercise with different degrees of intensity and use up insulin and food differently. So the intensity and timing of exercise and their effect on the blood sugar level must be considered.

The timing of exercise should be convenient but also it should, if possible, take place when it is most effective in controlling the blood sugar level. For example, afternoon exercising (between three and five p.m.), when the blood sugar level is high, may bring the level down. All diabetics, both insulin- and non-insulin-dependent, must be alert to the possibility of hypoglycaemic reactions (insulin reactions). Exercise should always be avoided when the blood sugar level is very high.

A patient may have to eat immediately before or after exercise – even during the exercise if hypoglycaemia occurs or is a recurrent problem. Exercise may decrease the insulin requirement, so it may be necessary to reduce the dose on the day of exercising. A doctor's advice on adjusting insulin dosage or meals in conjunction with exercise is important.

Selecting the Right Exercise
Vigorous exercises that use up more calories lead to better conditioning and physical fitness. Running, contact sports and tennis are examples but they are not possible for every-body, and the doctor's advice is important. The aim is to use up at least 100 to 200 calories in each exercise period. Table 1 outlines approximate calorie expenditure for various activi-ties. And remember – to be effective exercise must be done regularly.

Ideally the exercise programme should increase the heart rate, promoting calorie expenditure and improving circula-tion and muscle conditioning. Ask your doctor to explain how to measure your heart rate and how to evaluate the effect of your exercise. Start gradually and work up to a minimum total of 90 aerobic minutes (see below) in three to five sessions a week. Each exercise session should last about 20–30 minutes. But do not overdo it. Always warm up before starting and warm down at the end.

Aerobic Exercise
Aerobic means 'with oxygen', and describes any sustained exercise that increases the heart rate. A good aerobic activity is one in which the large muscle masses of the body are used. Jogging, cycling, swimming and aerobic dancing are good examples. They burn calories, tone up muscles and, if per-

TABLE 1. CALORIES EXPENDED IN VARIOUS ACTIVITIES
(APPROX)

Activity	Calories per hour
Moderate:	
Cycling (5½ mph)	210
Exercise cycle (5 mph)	210
Walking (2½ mph)	210
Canoeing (2½ mph)	230
Bowling	270
Rowing (2½ mph)	300
Swimming (¼ mph)	300
Walking (3¾ mph)	300
Badminton	350
Horse riding (trotting)	350
Volleyball	350
Ice-skating or roller-skating	350
Vigorous:	
Tennis, doubles	360
Tennis, singles	420
Aerobic dancing	420
Water-skiing	480
Hill-climbing (100 feet/hour)	490
Skiing, downhill	600
Jogging (5 mph)	600
Squash or handball, practice	600
Running (5½ mph)	650
Cycling (13 mph)	660
Scull rowing (race)	840
Running (10 mph)	900

Source: Adapted from the President's Council on
Physical Fitness in Sports, Washington, DC, and the
American Diabetes Guide to Good Living, New York,
American Diabetes Association, 1982.

formed correctly, strengthen the heart and blood vessels.
There are three essentials for aerobic conditioning:

1. Frequency: the activity must be done at least three
   times a week, preferably on alternate days.

2. Intensity: the heart rate must reach a target of 70 to 80 per cent of the maximum attainable heart rate.
3. Duration: the exercise must be maintained at the target heart rate for at least 20 minutes.

TABLE 2. RECOMMENDED SNACKS BEFORE EXERCISE

Type of exercise	Example*	If blood sugar (mmol/L) is:	Increase food intake by:	Suggested foods
Moderate intensity, short duration	Walking 1 mile or leisure cycling for less than ½ hr	4 or above	Not necessary	
		Less than 4	10–15 g of carbohydrate	Sandwich or snack bar
Moderate intensity	Tennis, swimming, jogging, leisure cycling, gardening, golfing, vacuum-cleaning for 1 hr	4–10	10–15 g of carbohydrate per hour of exercise	Sandwich or snack bar
		Less than 4	25–30 g of carbohydrate prior to exercise; 10–15 g per hour of exercise	Sandwich, biscuits or snack bar, with milk or juice
		10–16	Not necessary to increase food	

* Prolonged exercise may require additional carbohydrate for up to 4 hours after exercise.

Type of exercise	Example*	If blood sugar (mmol/L) is:	Increase food intake by:	Suggested foods
		16 or above	Do not exercise until blood sugar is under better control†	
Strenuous	Football, hockey, racquetball or basketball, strenuous cycling or swimming	4–10	25–30 g of carbohydrate, depending on intensity and duration	Sandwich or snack bar with milk or juice
		Less than 4	50 g of carbohydrate; monitor blood sugar carefully	20–25 g of carbohydrate from a non-concentrate source (i.e., Red Section of *Countdown*) plus sandwich or snack bar with milk or juice
		4–16	10–15 g of carbohydrate per hour of exercise	
		16 or above	Do not exercise until blood sugar is under better control†	

† When the blood sugar level is 16 mmol/L or more, exercise may cause it to rise further.

Target heart rate is determined by the maximum attainable heart rate, and this is related to age. A doctor's advice should be obtained on setting the target and learning how to measure it. Exercising at less than 70 per cent of one's maximum heart rate will not provide a heavy enough workload for aerobic conditioning, while more than 85 per cent will lead to fatigue and injury, so one must pace oneself, checking the heart rate periodically during the exercise:

1. About two minutes after starting.
2. Midway through the activity.
3. After it is completed.

If the heart rate is above the target rate the pace of the exercise should be slowed. If it is lower, and there are no symptoms of over-exertion, the pace can be increased slightly.

Special Precautions for Insulin-dependent Diabetics
The insulin-dependent diabetic should choose an enjoyable exercise, then find out how it affects his or her blood sugar level by careful self monitoring. Adjustments in the timing of meals and insulin doses should be based on the doctor's advice.

A good time for exercise is an hour or two before a meal. It should not be done immediately after insulin is taken or when insulin is at peak effectiveness. Blood sugar level should be checked before exercising and a snack eaten according to the guidelines in Table 2.

The insulin-dependent diabetic should always eat before any *extra* exercise – that is, exercise that is not part of normal routine – of whatever kind. Insulin must never be skipped except on doctor's orders, and the injections should preferably be at a site not affected by the exercise.

Select proper equipment. Shoes and clothing should be light and cool, the shoes giving good support to joints and muscles. Exercise should be avoided during illness, when ketoacids are in the urine, or after a large meal. Do not take alcohol just before or after exercise, try to avoid temperature extremes and drink enough water to replace fluid lost by sweating.

Allow 10 to 15 minutes for a warm-up and the same for cooling down. Try to breathe out during the effort cycle. If any pain is felt in the chest, teeth, jaw, or arm, or if the heart rate becomes irregular, stop the exercise at once and report the symptoms to your doctor. Try to avoid exercising alone, and carry glucose tablets or some simple form of sugar for use in case of hypoglycaemic reaction ('hypo').

All-day activities, such as skiing or backpacking, call for careful planning of insulin doses and meal times. Be rather *over*prepared, with extra food and easy-to-carry carbohydrates such as glucose tablets or gel in case of hypoglycaemic reaction. Remember, hypoglycaemia is possible for several hours after the exercise.

Guidelines for Non-insulin-dependent Diabetics
For non-insulin-dependent diabetics regular exercise combined with weight loss may be all that is needed to control blood sugar levels, and those on medication often find that doses can be cut down or even dropped once exercise becomes part of their regular routine.

Before starting any exercise programme more strenuous than walking, discuss it with your doctor. Don't overdo it. Work up gradually to the desired level of activity. Always warm up before a session and cool down after it. Have a doctor explain how to measure your heart rate and recognize any signs of an adverse effect. If you feel pain in the chest, teeth, jaw, or arm or your heartbeat becomes irregular, stop the activity immediately. Report these symptoms to your doctor.

6. Nutrition

Goals of Dietary Management
The underlying goals of all diets for diabetics are: (1) to provide enough calories to promote growth in children; (2) to maintain ideal body weight in lean adults or decrease weight in overweight patients; (3) to reduce breakdown of body fat (ketoacidosis) and body protein; (4) to avoid hyperglycaemia (high blood sugar level) and hypoglycaemia (low blood sugar level); and (5) to control blood levels of lipids, cholesterol and triglycerides.

To achieve this, three basic dietary principles must be considered. The diet must be balanced, i.e. containing the right amounts of nutrients to promote and maintain good health. Food intake must be distributed over the day so as to avoid fluctuations in blood sugar level, the distribution and number of calories consumed being consistent from day to day. The diet must be flexible and palatable enough to be followed willingly and adaptable to changing situations – for example, when travelling, eating out, attending a party, or ill. The individual who spends some time initially learning about his or her diet will be able to adapt it to most circumstances without disrupting treatment.

Doctors and dietitians consider many factors when developing a dietary plan. We discuss the main ones below.

Calories
Total daily calorie intake is fundamental to the programme. Usually an allowance of 12 to 15 calories per pound of ideal

weight is adequate to maintain body weight. However, previous intake is an essential guide.

Intake should be spread as evenly as possible over the day. Generally three to six meals are recommended, depending on the individual's specific treatment programme and lifestyle. Diabetics being treated by diet alone usually need only three meals a day, unless a bedtime snack is also desired. Those on oral medication usually need only three meals a day, but a bedtime snack may be added if the patient wishes or to avoid a low blood sugar level during the night.

Most diabetics taking insulin need four to six meals a day, depending on their lifestyle and the type of insulin and schedule of doses. The timing of meals for insulin-dependent diabetics is very important because carbohydrate intake must be timed to correspond with the circulating insulin level. If a meal is skipped or not enough food is eaten there will be too little sugar circulating and hypoglycaemia can occur.

The three basic nutrients – protein, fat and carbohydrate – all supply calories. Protein and carbohydrates supply 4 calories per gram and fat supplies 9 per gram. About 50 per cent of daily calorie intake should be in the form of carbohydrate, and of this 50 to 70 per cent should be complex carbohydrate like whole grains, beans, pasta, rice, vegetables and fruit. The remaining calories are provided by protein and fat. Usually, fat should contribute no more than 30–35 per cent of the total calorie intake, and for a patient with cardiovascular disease fat intake may be even lower.

Each meal should be a mix of carbohydrate, protein and fat. Because the timing of meals, distribution of calories and type of food consumed affect the blood sugar and insulin levels, it is very important that a personal meal plan be developed to meet the patient's particular needs. Once the meal plan is set up it should be followed as regularly and consistently as possible.

For overweight patients, the calorie level of a diet is designed to bring about weight loss without loss of muscle. An ideal weight-loss diet produces a progressive loss of 1 to 3 pounds each week and allows for developing new eating patterns that will enable the patient to keep the weight down. Fad diets or menu plans may lead to more rapid weight loss but inevitably it is body protein and water that are lost, not body fat. Therefore, the weight loss is only temporary. A slower approach will lead to more permanent weight loss. Losing weight and keeping it off are not easy to do alone. A weight control group can lend one support.

A useful approach to weight control is behaviour modification. This is based on the notion that to lose weight and keep it off one must change the habits that encourage eating, and the easiest way to do this is to replace them with new habits that permit weight control. Here are specific steps that can help:

1. Chew your food slowly.
2. Never shop for food when you are hungry.
3. Always make out a shopping list in advance. Do not add to it during shopping.
4. Do not leave food on the table.
5. Always sit down to eat.
6. Restrict eating to one or two places such as the kitchen and dining-room.
7. Never eat while engaging in another activity such as watching television.
8. Examine your own individual eating pattern so that you can identify problems and make the necessary changes. It helps to keep a diary of when and where you eat and in what circumstances – for example, frustration, anger, boredom, hunger, time of day.
9. Do not keep high-calorie foods or snacks around, but keep low-calorie foods available as snacks.
10. Get your family to help you in changing your eating habits.
11. Do not skip meals.
12. Work out a reward system for weight-loss.

13. Develop a slimming plan and continually evaluate and update it.
14. Make only one change at a time.
15. Make a personal commitment to weight loss.
16. If possible, institute a regular exercise programme.
17. Never drive when you can walk.
18. Use stairs instead of lifts.
19. Take a walk or exercise at times when you usually eat a snack.
20. Do not be afraid to make more than one trip up the stairs each day.

Carbohydrates

There are two types of carbohydrates. Refined carbohydrates, such as sugar and simple starches, are quickly absorbed into the body. Unrefined carbohydrates, such as whole grains, vegetables and pasta, must be broken down (digested) before they can be absorbed, so they are later and slower in increasing the blood sugar level.

Refined carbohydrates are more quickly absorbed when they are the only food eaten and absorbed more slowly when eaten as part of a mixed meal containing unrefined carbohydrate, protein and fat. This blunts the peaks in blood sugar levels after meals. Fat and protein also tend to reduce the speed at which the stomach empties, which in turn reduces blood sugar peaks after meals. This makes it possible to include some refined carbohydrates in the diet, but *only* when they are consumed as part of a mixed meal. This interaction also makes it possible to eat commercial foods which include small amounts of concentrated carbohydrates, such as sugar, in recipes that also include other carbohydrates, protein and fat. See the list of foods on page 88 which will help you in meal planning.

Previously it was thought that carbohydrates with the same chemical structure had the same effect on blood sugar levels. Now it is known that carbohydrate consumed in liquid form, like orange juice, is absorbed more rapidly than the same carbohydrate in solid form, e.g. a whole fresh orange. Absorption of carbohydrate is also affected by the way in which food is processed and cooked. Foods containing complex carbohydrates do not affect the blood sugar level in the same way. For example, bread, potato and rice increase the blood sugar level more than bran, oatmeal, peas, beans, pasta, peanuts and ice-cream do.

Because most people do not eat a meal consisting only of potatoes or rice it is difficult to predict exactly what will result from a given meal. When a meal is a mix of nutrients, each one influences the absorption of all the others.

Fibre
Dietary fibre is the part of plant foods that contains indigestible and unabsorbable carbohydrate. There are several general types, all with different physical properties and therefore producing different effects when consumed. Some increase gastric bulk and help food to pass more quickly through the gastro-intestinal tract. Others bind cholesterol, thereby lowering the blood cholesterol level. High-fibre diets help you reduce calorie intake because they contribute to a feeling of fullness and satisfaction. A high-fibre diet can reduce the insulin needs of some diabetics. The value of fibre is that it slows down absorption of sugar without increasing calorie intake.

Fresh fruits, vegetables and whole grain products are important sources of fibre. Products such as methyl cellulose, pectin and guar can be incorporated in the diet to increase fibre content. Bran provides a good source of cellulose, and fruits provide a good source of pectin. Guar is a powder used to thicken soups or in making gelatine desserts, bread and biscuits. But guar tends to impart a heavy texture to bread or biscuits and must be used judiciously. Do not use without first consulting your doctor.

A high-fibre diet is one containing about 20–25 g of fibre –

ideally from natural whole foods – per 1,000 calories daily. A diet containing 30 g or more of fibre per 1,000 calories is most likely to be associated with better blood sugar control.

Dietary fibre makes for good bowel movement, but large amounts can cause abdominal cramps and diarrhoea, so it is best to build up the amount in the diet gradually over a period. High-fibre diets may be inappropriate for patients with gastric problems and for some elderly people. Before greatly increasing the amount of fibre in your diet, check with your doctor.

A food that is high in fibre is usually one in its whole, natural state rather than processed: for example, whole-grain cereal products like bran or oat cereal, or wholemeal bread instead of white bread; fresh, whole fruit in their skins instead of juices and tinned fruit; fresh vegetables, lentils, dried beans; whole barley, brown rice, nuts and seeds are also excellent sources of fibre.

Cooking Hints for Using Whole-grain Products

Always stir whole-grain flour well before sifting. The bran remains in the sifter, so put it back in the flour mixture.

When replacing ordinary flour in a recipe with whole-grain flour, more liquid, extra yeast and longer kneading will probably be needed. One-third to half of the refined flour in any recipe can usually be replaced with whole-grain flour without changing the taste significantly.

Brush whole-grain bread with a little melted margarine while still hot to keep the crust from getting too hard.

Brown rice takes longer to cook; follow the directions on the packet. To cook a mixture of brown and white rice start with the brown rice and add the white later.

Follow package directions for sorting and rinsing peas and beans before cooking them.

Using Sugar and Sugar Substitutes

So long as the overall diet contains reasonable quantities of natural fibre and a good balance of protein, fat and unrefined carbohydrates, small amounts of foods pre-sweetened by the manufacturer are permissible. For instance, a high-fibre breakfast cereal that includes sugar or glucose in its ingredients is actually preferable to a more refined cereal without sugar. Nevertheless, to achieve optimum control the amount and timing of such foods must be carefully regulated. Presweetened foods are best taken as part of a whole meal, not at snack times. The lists on pages 51–9 and booklets such as *Countdown*, published by the British Diabetic Association, will help in menu-planning.

This new flexibility has broadened the range of foods available to diabetics, but the British Diabetic Association still recommends that whenever possible diabetics and their families should avoid using simple sugars. The many sugar substitutes that can be used in preparing food are helpful here. Useful for sweetening beverages, fruit and milk-based desserts are the various tablet and liquid sweeteners based upon saccharin, acesulfame K and aspartame. They add no extra calories to the diet and so are suitable for all diabetics, including those on weight reduction programmes. Obviously it is best to lose one's 'sweet tooth', so recipes in this book avoid the unnecessary use of sweetening agents. If they are needed they should be only those based on saccharin, acesulfame K or aspartame. Sweeteners containing sugar, lactose (milk sugar), sorbitol or fructose (fruit sugar) will add calories, and sometimes extra carbohydrate, to a recipe. When devising recipes you may occasionally need the physical properties of sugar – such as its ability to bulk or to preserve – rather than its sweetening power. At such times, bulk substitutes like those based on sorbitol with saccharin, or fructose may be necessary. Individual advice will vary, but non-obese diabetics are generally permitted such substitutes provided that their total daily intake of one or of a combination does not exceed 25 grams, a scant ounce. At present these substitutes are thought to offer some advantages over sugar, but future research may show that sugar (in small quantities) in home baking may be acceptable in a diabetic diet.

Sodium and Salt

If you want to cut down on your sodium intake, watch your consumption of table salt, which is about 40 per cent sodium. Sodium is found in many other food items, and is widely used as a preservative in various processed food products. Check labels carefully for salt and sodium-containing additives. If either is listed as the first or second ingredient avoid the product. Other sources of sodium are chemically softened water, some toothpastes, baking powder, baking soda, mono-sodium glutamate, meat sauces, flavouring condiments, kosher foods and many convenience foods.

Take the salt-cellar off the table and gradually reduce the amount of salt used in cooking. As your sodium intake decreases so will your taste for salt, and you will begin to enjoy the natural taste of food.

Protein

Protein is used by the body to build and maintain the tissues. It also contributes calories to meet energy requirements. Good sources are meat, milk, poultry, fish, cheese, eggs, peas and beans. Diabetic diets are planned to provide enough protein for the patient's nutritional needs. There is no benefit in extra protein. Much of it contains unhealthy saturated fat and it increases the cost of the diet.

Peas and beans are an excellent source of protein. However, the protein is 'incomplete' and does not contain all the protein components needed by the body. If you plan to use peas and beans as a main source of protein, the missing components must be added in the form of whole-grain products, nuts, seeds and dairy products. People not used to eating large amounts of peas and beans can suffer intestinal bloating and wind from them.

7. Planning Meals

Varying the Foods You Eat

Having your daily calories or carbohydrate regulated does not mean you must have the same foods each day. This would be extremely boring and probably impossible to follow. For this reason dietitians have developed food lists that itemize calorie and carbohydrate content. Once you know the amount of carbohydrate or calories you can have at each meal or for the whole day, you can use the lists to plan interesting and varied meals and, of course, develop your own recipes. It is clear from the previous chapters that not only the right amounts of carbohydrate and/or calories are important but that enough fibre and protein must be provided and excessive fat avoided. In the following lists foods that are major sources of fibre or fat are highlighted so that you may include more of the former and fewer of the latter when planning meals.

Using the Lists

Your diet prescription will have been worked out by your doctor and dietitian. For those on carbohydrate-controlled diets the amounts will be based upon approximate calorie need, half of the calories coming from the carbohydrate prescription (see following table). You should ensure that at least two-thirds of your carbohydrate choices are also good fibre sources. To keep your fat and calorie intake under control, keep fat sources to a minimum.

In the first list you will find foods that must be fitted into your carbohydrate allowance. When eaten in the amounts described each food will provide 10 grams of carbohydrate, which you may know as one carbohydrate exchange, portion or ration. If you have been advised to have, say, four exchanges or 40 grams of carbohydrate you can choose any four items from the list or, if you particularly like one kind of food, four times the amount of food stated to provide your allowance of 40 g (or exchanges).

HOW MUCH CARBOHYDRATE?

On 1000 calories a day, aim at 120 grams carbohydrate (CHO)
On 1200 calories a day, aim at 150 grams carbohydrate (CHO)
On 1500 calories a day, aim at 180 grams carbohydrate (CHO)
On 1800 calories a day, aim at 220 grams carbohydrate (CHO)
On 2000 calories a day, aim at 250 grams carbohydrate (CHO)
On 2200 calories a day, aim at 270 grams carbohydrate (CHO)
On 2500 calories a day, aim at 300 grams carbohydrate (CHO)
On 2800 calories a day, aim at 350 grams carbohydrate (CHO)
On 3000 calories a day, aim at 380 grams carbohydrate (CHO)

In the second list are foods that are not carbohydrate sources. These can be selected to accompany your carbohydrate choices, but you should be guided by their calorie content and the symbols on the high-fat foods with regard to frequency and quantities. If you are on insulin and on a carbohydrate-controlled diet but are having difficulty controlling your weight you should make a particular point of selecting from the lower-calorie choices and, if possible, check your calorie intake regularly. Readers on calorie-controlled diets should ensure that at least half their calorie intake comes from foods in the carbohydrate-containing list and that as many good fibre choices as possible are included daily.

Foods containing negligible amounts of calories are on the third list. Those which are low in calories and carbohydrate and so not usually counted when eaten as meal accompaniments are on the fourth list.

It is important that you eat a balanced diet, with all necessary nutrients – vitamins, minerals and trace elements as well as protein, fat, carbohydrate, fibre and total calories.

While many foods seem to have similar carbohydrate or calorie values they differ in nutrient-content, so it is important to choose a wide variety across the week. At the end of the lists you will find a sample day's meals selected from the lists. You can, of course, make use of commercially prepared foods (details of nutritional content may appear on the packaging or be found in the British Diabetic Association's publication *Countdown*), or recipes from cookbooks like this one, in which nutritional information is given with the recipes.

Getting to Know the Portion Sizes
You should quickly become used to judging the portion sizes that will provide the carbohydrate and/or calories that you need. In the lists, as well as weights, homely measures are given, and you should try to use them whenever possible and not rely on scales or other measuring devices. Obviously you must check your judgement against an actual weight now and then, but don't be a slave to the scales.

Calculating Recipes
As well as using everyday foods, commercial foods and special recipes in cookbooks, in time you will probably want to develop your own recipes. Once you know the ingredients in a recipe you can use the food lists to work out available carbohydrate and calories. A sample recipe calculation using the lists is given below.

HOW TO CALCULATE A RECIPE
Cheese Scones – makes 8 scones

Food	Weight	Carbohydrate	Calories
Wholemeal flour	100 g	65 g	325
Low-fat spread	50 g	—	270
Edam cheese	25 g	—	75
Parmesan cheese	25 g	—	100
Skimmed milk	200 ml	10 g	70
Baking powder	2 teaspoons	—	—
Salt	¼ teaspoon	—	—
Totals for 8 scones		75 g	840

Therefore each scone is
approximately 10 g CHO and 105 calories

FOOD-VALUE LISTS FOR USE IN DIABETIC DIETS

LIST 1

In the following list all spoon measurements are assumed to have been
made using standard household measuring spoons.

Food	Approximate measure	Approximate weight of food in grams containing 10 grams carbohydrate	Calorie content
Starchy Foods			
Arrowroot/custard powder/cornflour	1 × 15 ml spoon (1 tablespoon)	10	35
*Barley/millet, whole	1 × 15 ml spoon (1 tablespoon)	10	40
Flour, plain, white	1½ × 15 ml spoon (1½ tablespoons)	10	40
self-raising, white	1½ × 15 ml spoon (1½ tablespoons)	10	45
*wholemeal/ wholewheat	2 × 15 ml spoons (2 tablespoons)	15	50
*Oats, uncooked	3 × 15 ml spoons (3 tablespoons)	15	60
Rice, white, uncooked	1 × 15 ml spoon (1 tablespoon)	10	45
*brown, uncooked	1 × 15 ml spoon (1 tablespoon)	10	40
Spaghetti, white, uncooked	6 long (19″) strands	10	45
*Spaghetti, wholewheat, uncooked	20 short (10″) strands	15	50
Sago/tapioca/semolina, uncooked	2 × 5 ml spoons (2 teaspoons)	10	35
White bread	1 small slice	20	50
*Wholemeal/wholewheat bread	1 small slice	25	50

(F) = High fat   * = High fibre

List 1 continued

Food	Approximate measure	Approximate weight of food in grams containing 10 grams carbohydrate	Calorie content
Biscuits/Crackers/Crispbreads			
Biscuits, plain	2	15	60
*Biscuits, digestive or wholemeal	1	15	70
Biscuits, cream or chocolate (F)	1	10	60
Crackers, plain	2	15	70
*Crispbreads, wholewheat	2	15	50
Breakfast Cereals			
*All-Bran	5 × 15 ml spoons (5 tablespoons)	20	50
*Bran Buds	(4 × 15 ml spoons (4 tablespoons)	20	50
Cornflakes	5 × 15 ml spoons (5 tablespoons)	10	40
*Muesli (unsweetened)	2 × 15 ml spoons (2 tablespoons)	15	50
*Muesli (sweetened)	2 × 15 ml spoons (2 tablespoons)	15	55
*Puffed Wheat	15 × 15 ml spoons (15 tablespoons)	15	50
Rice Krispies	6 × 15 ml spoons (6 tablespoons)	10	40
Special K	8 × 15 ml spoons (8 tablespoons)	15	50
*Spoonsize Cubs	12–14	—	45
*Weetabix	1	—	60
*Weetaflakes	4 × 15 ml spoons (4 tablespoons)	15	50

Fruit Juices (unsweetened)
The carbohydrate values will vary slightly from one fruit to another and according to the time of year.

Apple/pineapple juice, unsweetened	6 × 15 ml spoons (6 tablespoons)	85	40

Grapefruit juice, unsweetened	8 × 15 ml spoons (8 tablespoons)	125	45
Orange juice, unsweetened	7 × 15 ml spoons (7 tablespoons)	100	40
Tomato juice, unsweetened	1 large glass	275	50
Fruits			
Apples, eating, whole	1 medium	110	50
cooking, whole	1 medium	125	55
stewed without sugar	6 × 15 ml spoons (6 tablespoons)	125	40
Apricots, fresh, whole	3 medium	160	40
*dried, raw	4 small	25	45
Bananas, with skin	5½″ in length	90	40
peeled	3½″ in length	50	40
*Blackberries, raw	10 × 15 ml spoons (10 tablespoons)	150	45
*Blackcurrants, raw	10 × 15 ml spoons (10 tablespoons)	150	45
Cherries, fresh, whole	12	100	40
*Currants, dried	2 × 15 ml spoons (2 tablespoons)	15	35
Damsons, raw, whole	7	120	40
Dates, fresh, whole	3 medium	50	40
*dried, without stones	3 small	15	40
Figs, fresh, whole	1	100	40
*dried	1	20	40
Grapes, whole	10 large	75	40
Guavas, fresh, flesh only	1	70	45
Kiwi	2 average	90	40
Mango, fresh, whole	⅓ of a large one	100	40
Melon, all types, weighed with skin	large slice	300	40
Nectarine, fresh, whole	1	90	40
Orange, fresh, whole	1 large	150	40
Paw-paw, fresh, whole	⅙ of a large one	80	50
Peach, fresh, whole	1 large	125	40
Pears, fresh, whole	1 large	130	40
Pineapple, fresh, no skin or core	1 thick slice	90	40

List 1 continued

Food	Approximate measure	Approximate weight of food in grams containing 10 grams carbohydrate	Calorie content
Plums, cooking, fresh, whole	4 medium	180	40
dessert, fresh, whole	2 large	110	40
Pomegranate, fresh, whole	1 small	110	40
*Prunes, dried, without stones	2 large	25	40
*Raisins, dried	2 × 15 ml spoons (2 tablespoons)	15	35
*Raspberries, fresh	12 × 15 ml spoons (12 tablespoons)	175	45
Strawberries, fresh	15 medium	160	40
*Sultanas, dried	2 × 15 ml spoons (2 tablespoons)	15	40
Tangerines, fresh, whole	2 large	175	40
Milk and Milk Products			
Milk, whole (F)	1 cup	200	130
skimmed	1 cup	200	70
semi-skimmed	1 cup	200	100
dried, skimmed	10 × 15 ml spoons (10 tablespoons)	20	70
evaporated (F)	6 × 15 ml spoons (6 tablespoons)	90	145
Yogurt, low fat, plain	1 small carton	150	80
Vegetables			
Beans, *baked	4 × 15 ml spoons (4 tablespoons)	75	55
*broad, boiled	10 × 15 ml spoons (10 tablespoons)	150	75
*dried, all types, raw	2 × 15 ml spoons (2 tablespoons)	20	55
Beetroot, cooked, whole	2 small	100	45

*Lentils, dry, raw	2 × 15 ml spoons (2 tablespoons)	20	60
Onions, raw	1 large	200	45
Parsnips, raw	1 small	90	45
*Peas, marrow fat or processed	7 × 15 ml spoons (7 tablespoons)	75	60
*Peas, dried, all types, raw	2 × 15 ml spoons (2 tablespoons)	20	60
Plantain, green, raw, peeled	small slice	35	40
Potatoes, raw	1 small egg-sized	50	45
boiled	1 small egg-sized	50	40
chips (weighed when cooked)	4–5 average chips	25	65
*jacket (weighed with skin)	1 small	50	45
mashed	1 small scoop	50	80
roast	½ medium	40	65
*Sweetcorn, canned or frozen	5 × 15 ml spoons (5 tablespoons)	60	45
*Sweetcorn, on the cob	½ medium cob	75	60
Sweet potato, raw, peeled	1 small slice	50	45

Manufactured Foods
A few typical manufactured foods are listed below. There are considerable variations from one brand to another. For accurate figures look on the package or in the British Diabetic Association publication *Countdown*.

Beefburgers, frozen (F)	3 small	75–100	450
Fish fingers	2	50	110
Ice-cream	1 scoop	50	90
Sausages (F)	2 thick	110	400
Soup	1 cup	200	115

LIST 2

The foods listed below contain a negligible amount of carbohydrate but their calorie content must not be forgotten when planning your meals.

Food	Approximate measure	Approximate weight of food in grams	Calorie content
Butter/margarine (F)	—	25	185
Low-fat spreads	—	25	95
Egg, medium, uncooked	1	55	80
Oil, vegetable (F)	1 × 15 ml spoon (1 tablespoon)	15	135
Cream, single (F)	small pot	150	320
double (F)	small pot	150	670
whipped (F)	small pot	150	500
Cheese			
Cheddar (F)	small matchbox size	25	100
Cottage	small pot	100	100
Edam (F)	small matchbox size	25	75
Parmesan (F)	3 × 15 ml spoons (3 tablespoons)	25	100
Processed (F)	1 slice	20	70
Quark	2 × 15 ml spoons (2 tablespoons)	25	25
Stilton (F)	small matchbox size	25	115
Meat			
Bacon, lean, grilled	1 rasher	25	75
lean, fried (F)	1 rasher	25	85
streaky, grilled (F)	1 rasher	25	105
streaky, fried (F)	1 rasher	25	125
Liver, raw	2 small slices	75	100–130
Meat, lean, raw	1 average helping	100	125
lean, cooked	1 average helping	100	160

fatty, raw (F)	1 average helping	100	410
Poultry, white meat, cooked	1 average helping	100	140
dark meat, cooked	1 average helping	100	155
Lamb cutlet, grilled (F)	1 medium	100	250
Pork chop, grilled (F)	1 medium	150	390
Corned beef (F)	2 slices	50	110
Fish			
Fish fillets, white, raw	1 average helping	100	80
fatty, raw	1 average helping	100	230
Shellfish, shelled	1 average helping	100	80–100
Tinned mackerel in tomato sauce	½ small can	100	130
Tinned tuna in brine	1 small can	100	100
Nuts and Seeds			
Almonds, shelled (F)	4 × 15 ml spoons (4 tablespoons)	50	280
Brazil nuts, shelled (F)	14 medium	50	310
Hazelnuts, shelled (F)	6 × 15 ml spoons (6 tablespoons)	50	190
Coconut, dried (F)	5 × 15 ml spoons (5 tablespoons)	25	150
Peanuts, roast (F)	1 small packet	25	145
*Sesame/sunflower seeds (F)	1 × 15 ml spoon (1 tablespoon)	25	140
Walnuts (F)	16 halves	50	130

LIST 3

These foods add negligible amounts of calories to your diet:

Clear soup/consommé
Coffee/tea/herbal tea
'Low calorie' or 'diabetic' soft drinks
Soda and spa waters
Herbs, spices, low-calorie sweeteners (e.g. acesulfame, aspartame, saccharin)

LIST 4

The following add very little carbohydrate or calories when eaten in normal portions. These do not need to be subtracted from your carbohydrate allowance and will not add more than 20–25 calories per serving:

Fruits

cranberries	gooseberries	lemons
loganberries	rhubarb	

Vegetables

artichokes	cabbage	lettuce	pumpkin
asparagus	carrots	marrow	radishes
aubergine	cauliflower	mushrooms	spinach
beans (runner)	celery	mustard and	spring onions
beansprouts	courgettes	cress	swede
broccoli	cucumber	okra (raw)	tomatoes (raw
Brussels	leeks	peas (fresh or	and canned)
sprouts		frozen)	turnip
		peppers	watercress

A TYPICAL DAY'S MEALS ON A 200 G CHO DIET (APPROXIMATELY 1600 CALORIES)
Distribution: 40   20   50   20   50   20

	Carbohydrate grams	Calories
Breakfast		
2 Weetabix	20	120
1 small banana	10	40
1 cup skimmed milk	10	70
Mid-morning		
1 digestive biscuit	10	70
1 fresh pear	10	40
Lunch		
Tuna (100 g)	neg	100
1 large jacket potato (150 g)	30	145
Salad (from List 4)	—	25
Sweetcorn (60 g)	10	45
Bowl of strawberries	10	40
Mid-afternoon		
1 wholemeal biscuit	10	70
Coffee made with semi-skimmed milk	10	100
Evening Meal		
Cooked lean meat (150 g)	—	240
Boiled potatoes (2 small)	20	80
Vegetables (from List 4)	—	25
Butter beans (40 g) boiled	20	110
1 carton low-fat plain yogurt	10	80

Bedtime

Wholemeal toast (50 g)	20	100
Low-fat spread (10 g)	—	40
Cheese (1 slice)	—	70
Coffee		
Totals	200 g	1610

Specialist Foods

There are prepared foods that make specialist claims including 'low-calorie', 'reduced calorie' and 'diabetic ranges'. Low-calorie items are useful for all diabetics as they can add only small quantities of calories and carbohydrate to the total diet. Those claiming 'reduced energy' may be helpful, but must be selected carefully and used as part of the diet plan. Under new legislation 'reduced energy' foods offer at least a 25 per cent saving in energy (calories), but they still provide significant amounts of energy and carbohydrate and so must be fitted into the diet plan.

Diabetic foods must not contain more calories or fat than ordinary foods but need not offer a calorie saving so they must be used very carefully by all diabetics, particularly those achieving control by weight-reduction. Legislation which became mandatory upon manufacturers in 1986 requires that all foods claiming to be suitable for diabetics must carry a warning that they are 'not suitable for overweight diabetics' unless they offer a 50 per cent reduction in calories.

Fat Intake

As noted earlier the British Diabetic Association recommends that total fat in the diet should not be more than 30–35 per cent of total calories in the diet plan. This is a reduction from the amount of fat eaten in a traditional diabetic diet and is in line with new thinking on the role of fat in heart disease. Heart disease has become the scourge of the civilized world and in many countries recommendations are being made to cut down fat intake in the belief that it may reduce the incidence of heart disease. Diabetics are at particular risk of developing cardiovascular disease, so they should be diligent in reducing their fat intake.

As well as reducing the total amount of fat eaten it is advised that less animal fat be eaten. Spreading fats and fats used in cooking should be from plant sources whenever possible, so polyunsaturated vegetable margarine and vegetable oils are preferable to hard fats.

It is thought that lower total fat intake plus reduced animal fats will cut down the levels of fat, particularly cholesterol, in the blood which, when high, seem to increase the risk of heart disease. If your blood cholesterol level remains high, despite reduced fat intake, your doctor may also advise reducing foods that contain cholesterol. This will involve eating a maximum of only 2–3 whole eggs a week, avoiding sea food and offal and making cream a rare treat. About half our fat intake comes from foods easily recognized as containing fat, the other half from foods in which the fat is less visible. When cooking and catering the following rules should be observed:

1. Use skimmed or semi-skimmed milk instead of full-fat milk. Semi-skimmed milk is quite acceptable in beverages and on cereals, and skimmed milk can be used in cooking.
2. Use such spreading fats as margarine and butter very sparingly, on only one slice of the bread for sandwiches, not at all if a moist filling is used. Try low-fat spreads if you have difficulty in being sparing with butter or margarine. If you have been told specifically to reduce cholesterol use 'polyunsaturated, low cholesterol' margarine rather than a low-fat spread, margarine or butter.
3. Eat poultry and fish rather than meat as they have a lower fat content. Limit meats such as beef, pork and lamb to a maximum of three or four times a week.
4. When cooking fattier cuts of meat, never add solid fat or oil. Try to skim off any fat from the stocks, stews and casseroles.

5. Grill rather than fry meat or meat products, and when cooking joints in the oven use a cooking rack so that the fat will drip away.

6. In recipes using cream try substituting yogurt or a skimmed-milk soft cheese.

7. Keep cheese intake to a minimum and substitute low-fat or reduced-fat cheese in place of full-fat, hard or cream cheese when possible.

8. Use vegetable oils rather than solid fat, the best ones being corn, sunflower, safflower and soya oil. As well as being better because unsaturated, in most cooking processes oil enables you to use less fat than you would using a solid kind. Even so, take care to add oil to a recipe only when necessary.

9. Make your own dressings for salads or vegetables, using yogurt or a selection of vinegars rather than oil-based dressings, or buy 'reduced-oil' or 'reduced-calorie' dressings in preference to full-fat ones.

8. Low-salt Meals

Sodium is a necessary component of the blood and an essential nutrient in our diet. It is found in varying amounts in almost everything we eat. The main source of sodium in the diet is table salt (sodium chloride) which is about 40 per cent sodium. A teaspoon of salt contains about 2 g of sodium. The average person consumes from 7 to 10 g of sodium per day, about 70 per cent contained naturally in food, the rest coming from added salt. Cured foods such as ham and bacon, condiments like sauces, pickles, steak sauce, mustard, ketchup and soy sauce, and many preservatives used in processing foods are major sources of sodium. Most fresh foods, particularly fruit and vegetables, contain lesser amounts of sodium. Indigestion tablets, some diet soft drinks, laxatives, cough medicines and some artificial sweeteners also contain significant amounts of sodium, so it is important to read labels carefully or to ask your dietitian about the sodium content in these products.

Most people can consume as much sodium as they want, but some cannot handle it and must be careful about their intake.

The taste for salt depends on how much one is exposed to it. Even people who salt their food heavily before tasting it will gradually lose their desire for salt if they stop using it. Recipes particularly high in sodium are marked with an asterisk (*).

Some Practical Suggestions
Start by taking the salt-cellar off the table and eliminating obviously salty foods from your diet – ham, bacon, steak

sauce, pre-salted potato crisps, canned or dried soups, salted salad dressings and condiments. Then gradually cut down the amount of salt used in cooking. Generally you will not have to use special low-sodium food products but, if you do, there are some available. Although most fresh fruit, vegetables, meats, poultry and fish are fine to use, when canned or frozen they may contain salt or a sodium preservative.

Check the ingredient list on all processed foods for the words salt, sodium, sodium chloride, soda, sodium compounds, or 'Na' (the chemical symbol for sodium). If one of these is among the first three ingredients listed you probably should avoid the product. Most cheeses are high in sodium but several low-sodium, low-fat cheeses are now available. These clearly indicate their salt and fat contents on the label.

Using Herbs and Spices

Learning to cook with less salt is easier if you learn to substitute for it the exciting tastes of herbs and spices. If you have never cooked with herbs and spices the following guidelines should be helpful.

1. Use herbs and spices sparingly. They should accentuate, not overpower, the flavour of the food.
2. When you start cooking with herbs use no more than a quarter of a teaspoon of dried herbs or three-quarters of a teaspoon of fresh herbs for a dish that serves four people. If you like the taste, you can always increase it the next time.
3. If you are preparing a recipe that is to be cooked for a long time, such as a soup or a stew, add the herbs during the last hour of cooking.
4. Add herbs to hamburgers, meat loaf and stuffing before cooking.
5. Sprinkle roasts, joints, steaks and chops with herbs before cooking.
6. Add herbs to vegetables, sauces and gravies while they are cooking.

7. Add herbs to cold foods – tomato juice, salad dressings and cottage cheese – several hours before serving. Storing the foods in the refrigerator for several hours or overnight will bring out the flavour of the herbs.
8. Heat and moisture bring out the fragrance and flavour of herbs. To add a subtle herb flavour to food, place the dried herbs in a tea strainer, dip the strainer into hot water for 20 seconds, drain the water and add the moistened herbs to the food.
9. To avoid having bits of the herb itself in the food, tie the herbs in a small piece of muslin and remove it before serving.
10. Marinating meat in a wine and herb mixture before cooking will greatly enhance its flavour.
11. To hasten the release of flavour, crush herbs in the palm of the hand before adding them to food.
12. When substituting fresh herbs for dried herbs, use three or four times as much of the fresh herbs.
13. Do not combine too many different herbs and spices in one dish or at one meal.

Cooking with Wine

Most of the alcohol used in cooking evaporates, leaving behind a wonderful taste but very few calories. Because only 1 or 2 tablespoons of alcohol per serving are used in most recipes the calories need not be calculated into the diet. The right amount of wine will enhance the flavour of the foods but, as the whole is only as good as its parts, use a good wine for cooking.

9. Guidelines for Special Situations

The regular diabetic diet is planned for the patient's regular pattern of activities, but special situations will arise – meals away from home, travel across time zones, occasional illness – and circumstances such as these call for adjustments in the routine. The information below is aimed at helping the patient to adjust to special situations. This information does not replace your doctor's advice and it is always wise to check with the doctor when you encounter a situation that has not been mentioned before. It is particularly important for the diabetic to stay in close touch with the doctor during illness.

Eating Away from Home
Being a diabetic is no hindrance to eating out. In fact, a diabetic diet is probably one of the easiest to follow in most restaurants. Once you know your meal plan and feel confident about estimating portions, you can choose safely from any menu.

Initially, try to select a meal that closely resembles your normal diet plan. It helps to carry a copy of the plan on you.

Because medication is taken at times related to food intake, it is important to eat at about the same times each day. When you plan to eat later than usual eat about one-third of your carbohydrate allowance at the ordinary time to tide you over. If dinner is to be very late eat your evening snack at your normal dinner time to stop the blood sugar level getting too low. If you are on a twice-daily insulin injection schedule, ask your doctor to explain the procedure for delaying your insulin injections if necessary.

Until you feel secure about your diet and about estimating portions, avoid dishes containing a mix of ingredients. Most restaurants will prepare simple food like grilled chicken, fish or meat. Ask for sauces, gravies, mayonnaise and dressings to be served separately so you can measure them accurately. Insist on fresh vegetables cooked without extra fat. Choose clear rather than cream soups and avoid fried foods and mixed casserole dishes.

Try fresh melon, fresh fruit cup, juice or broth as your appetizer, and fresh fruit for dessert. If you cannot live without a sweet dessert, you can occasionally order plain vanilla ice-cream (one scoop is equal to 10 g of carbohydrate).

To control your fat intake, avoid butter, and trim the fat and skin from poultry and meat.

Here are some ideas to help you choose a meal from a restaurant menu. Remember, the portion sizes are important and should conform as closely as possible to the meal plan. On a low-salt diet, avoid items marked * and ask for your food to be cooked without added salt.

Breakfasts

Cereal – ask for wholemeal or high-fibre cereal such as Shredded Wheat, Weetabix, Branflakes, All-Bran, muesli or porridge.

Bread – ask for wholemeal bread, or brown if this is not available.

Crispbreads – these are usually wholemeal, such as Ryvita.

Fruit juice – ask for unsweetened.

Cooked items – ask for poached or scrambled eggs rather than fried.

Avoid sausages* which are very fatty, but an occasional small helping of bacon* is permissible. Bulk out the meal with extra portions of tomatoes or mushrooms. Ask for unbuttered toast and use the spreading fat (if necessary) as sparingly as possible.

Midday and Evening Meals
Choose fruit juice or soup to start. Avoid cream soups, and choose a vegetable soup if possible. Melon or grapefruit are also useful starters and pâté or seafood cocktail* can be selected if you are not on a weight-loss diet.

Main Courses. Any meat, fish or poultry dish. Choose larger pieces of fried fish rather than scampi, whitebait, etc., which absorb more fat. Pastry dishes such as pies and puddings should be avoided as much as possible.

Accompaniments. Choose at least two accompanying vegetables and ask for jacket or mashed potatoes in preference to chips.

Desserts
Far from a necessity, but plain ice-cream, fresh fruit salad or a small helping of cheesecake is better than a heavy pudding or pastry.

Accompanying Beverages
Drink coffee without cream, tea or lemon tea. Choose dry wines and have no more than one or two glasses throughout the whole meal. A dry sherry, dry aperitif or half-pint of beer/lager can be drunk before the meal.

Eating in Ethnic Restaurants
When eating in an ethnic restaurant, you have to be well versed in your diet so as to recognize the ingredients in various dishes. Estimate as closely as possible the carbohydrate content of the dish that interests you. It is better to err on the side of overestimating than underestimating.

Fast Foods
There is no reason why a diabetic should not be able to enjoy a take-away meal or a quick snack. Fast food outlets generally

offer very standard portions and the approximate guide below
is sufficiently accurate for *occasional* use.

GUIDE TO FAST FOODS AND TAKE-AWAYS

MENU ITEM	Approximate content of carbohydrate, grams	Calories
Fish in batter	10–15	400–500
Chips (average portion from chip shop)	40–50	300–400
Chinese or Indian boiled rice (average portion)	80–90	350–400
Chinese fried rice (average portion)	80	600–700
Chinese chow mein (average portion)	50	250–300
Indian pilau rice	70–80	700–800
BURGERS (all figures include bun, relish, etc.)		
McDonalds		
Hamburger	30	260
Cheeseburger	30	300
Quarter Pounder	35	420
Quarter Pounder with Cheese	40	500
Big Mac	50–55	560
Fillet of fish	35	420
French fries, regular	35	290
French fries, large	50	390
Wendy's		
Quarter Pounder	35	470
Quarter Pounder with Cheese	35	580
Half Pounder	35	670
Half Pounder with Cheese	40	800
Triple	35	850
Triple with Cheese	35	1040
Chilli-burger	20	230
Chilli-burger with Cheese	25	330
Junior Hamburger	30	300
Junior Hamburger with Cheese	30	320
French fries, regular	40	330
Wimpy		
Hamburger (white bun)	30	240
Quarter Pounder (wheatmeal bun)	40	500

Quarter Pounder with Cheese		
(wheatmeal bun)	40	550
Half Pounder (wheatmeal bun)	40	800
Cheeseburger (white bun)	30	290
Kingsize (white bun)	30	400
Bacon-in-a-Bun (white bun)	30	280
Chicken-in-a-Bun (white bun)	45	430
Bacon and Egg-in-a-Bun (white bun)	30	420
OTHER DISHES		
Fish and Chips	45	490
Wimpy Grill	40	520
Wimpy Special Grill	40	670
Quarter Pounder Special Grill	40	700
International Grill	40	660
Chips	40	290

Eating on Aircraft

Most airlines offer a variety of meals to meet special religious or other dietary needs. Notify the reservations personnel when booking and remind the airline by letter. Because diabetic needs vary it is *essential* that you specify the kinds and amounts of foods needed for each meal in advance of your flight so that preparation can be made. When you check in mention that you have ordered a special meal. It is a good idea to carry some food with you on a trip in case of delays or mix-ups. Let the steward know when you have to eat so that your meal is not delayed.

Even if there is some problem you should be able to choose suitable food from the standard airline fare.

Eating at the Home of a Friend

Dinner at a friend's home need pose no problem if you tell your hosts in advance that you are a diabetic and must watch your diet. This will save embarrassment for both of you. They can plan the menu accordingly, and it will relieve you from being pressed to eat 'just a little more'. Hosts will understand if you ask for smaller portions or refuse dessert. Planning ahead will avoid unnecessary problems.

Alcohol

Alcohol is an excellent low-calorie, low-salt way to flavour food when cooking. The calories do not have to be allowed for in the diet if only small amounts of alcohol are used. Usually only 1 or 2 tbsp per serving is added in cooking, and the alcohol evaporates when it is heated. The remaining calories are from carbohydrate or protein contained in the drink.

An *occasional* cocktail or glass of wine is usually permissible for diabetics. But discuss it with your doctor first and find out exactly how much alcohol you may safely drink. Drink only in moderation and never on an empty stomach. Drink slowly, and avoid sugary or sweet drinks. If you are on a calorie-controlled diet, remember to count the calories and adjust your meal plan accordingly. *Diabetics taking insulin are advised not to substitute alcoholic drinks for their food carbohydrate allowance.* Moderate amounts of alcohol can be taken in addition to the normal carbohydrate allowance. *Insulin-dependent diabetics should never drink and drive or undertake other tasks that would be potentially dangerous if hypoglycaemia should occur.*

Travelling Across Time Zones

Travelling by air across time zones can pose a problem for the diabetic, and you should always ask your doctor for specific instructions on the timing of your medication. In general diabetics may take meals and insulin according to the time of day they arrive at their destination. Seek the advice of your doctor about specific changes you may need to make if you are taking insulin or an oral medication.

Illness

When an illness occurs, such as an upset stomach, sore throat or bad cold, it is still necessary to maintain your carbohydrate intake and drug doses, though you may have no appetite or are vomiting. If you cannot take solid food but can tolerate liquids you can maintain your calories with sweetened juices and soft drinks. In this way you will meet your energy needs and provide adequate carbohydrate to balance insulin action. When you are ill stay in close touch with your doctor for advice on diabetes management. Blood and urine sugar levels should be checked more frequently, usually every four to six hours, and you should always test for ketoacids in the urine. If control of a fever or cough is necessary, any standard remedy, such as aspirin and sugar-free cough syrup, can be used. Sugar-free medications are always to be preferred. In the event of hypoglycaemic reaction, the hormone glucagon may be necessary.

Insulin should never be stopped during an illness, regardless of decreased appetite or nausea and vomiting. Your doctor will help you adjust the dosage as necessary. Usually more, not less, insulin is needed during an acute illness. If persistent vomiting occurs, the blood sugar remains over 22 mmol/L and the urine ketoacid test remains positive despite the best efforts at control, it will probably be necessary to go into hospital.

Try to eat small amounts frequently, and take water, clear broth, tea and other fluids to replace lost salt and water. Sip sweet fizzy drinks or fruit juices every hour or so. Your need for insulin may increase during illness. Consult your doctor if you are ill for more than a day and unable to maintain your normal routine.

Meal Planning During Illness

Your diet may need to be modified during a period of illness. If you cannot eat your regular diet, replace the carbohydrate content with sweetened drinks and soft sweetened foods. Use the following list to provide a regular carbohydrate intake. It will probably not be necessary to have your full carbohydrate allowance, but aim to have at least half to three-quarters of your normal intake across the whole day. This might be more palatable divided equally as snacks every two hours rather than in your usual distribution.

Fluids to provide 10 g of carbohydrate	*Amount to be taken*
Coke or Pepsi, 1 wine glass	100 ml/4 fl oz
Fruit juices (natural, unsweetened), 1 wine glass	100 ml/4 fl oz
Lemonade or similar carbonated drink	150 ml/5 fl oz
Lucozade or similar glucose drink	50 ml/2 fl oz
Milk, 1 cup	200 ml/7 fl oz
Soup (thickened creamed – e.g. chicken), 1 cup	200 ml/7 fl oz
Soup (tomato, tinned), ½ cup	100 ml/4 fl oz

Foods to provide 10 g of carbohydrate	
Drinking chocolate, Horlicks, Ovaltine or similar malted drink	2 heaped teaspoonsful
Glucose tablets	3 tablets
Honey, jam or syrup	2 level teaspoonsful
Ice-cream (plain), 1 scoop or small brickette	50 g/2 oz
Natural yogurt, 1 pot	150 g/5 oz

Other useful carbohydrate-containing foods	*Carbohydrate content*
Build-up (Carnation), 1 envelope	25 g
Slender (Carnation), 1 envelope	20 g
Sweetened fruit yogurt, 1 pot (150 g/5 fl oz)	25–30 g

Glossary*

Acidosis
Too much acid in the body, for a diabetic usually ketoacidosis. See: Ketoacidosis.

Amino acids
The 'building blocks' of the proteins, main materials of the body's cells. Insulin is a protein comprising 51 linked amino acids.

Anti-diabetic agent
A substance that helps a diabetic to control the glucose (sugar) level in the blood so that the body works as it should. See: Insulin; Oral hypoglycaemic agents.

Arteries
Large blood vessels carrying blood from the heart to other parts of the body. Arteries are thicker, with stronger and more elastic walls than veins. See: Blood vessels.

Arteriosclerosis
Thickening and hardening of the walls of the arteries. In one type of arteriosclerosis fat builds up inside the walls and slows the blood flow. This often occurs in long-term diabetics.

Artificial endocrine pancreas
An artificial device that monitors glucose (sugar) in the blood and releases the exact amounts of insulin for the body's needs.

---

* Adapted from *The Diabetes Dictionary*, The National Diabetes Information Clearinghouse, National Institute of Arthritis, Diabetes, and Digestive and Kidney Diseases, National Institutes of Health, Bethesda, Maryland, 1984.

This is a large bedside machine, also called an 'artificial beta cell'.

Aspartame
An artificial low-calorie sweetener for use instead of sugar.

Atherosclerosis
A build-up of fat in the walls of large and medium-sized arteries which may slow down or stop the flow of blood. The disease can occur in long-term diabetics.

Beta cells
Cells in the islets of Langerhans of the pancreas which make and release insulin to control the level of glucose (sugar) in the blood. See: Insulin.

Biguanides
A group of drugs which lower the glucose (sugar) level in the blood. See: Oral hypoglycaemic agents.

Blood glucose
The main sugar made by the body from food's three elements – proteins, fats and carbohydrates – but mostly from carbohydrates. Glucose is the chief source of energy for living cells and is carried to them by the bloodstream, but they cannot use it without the help of insulin.

Blood glucose monitoring
A way of testing how much glucose (sugar) is in the blood. A drop of blood from the tip of a finger or an earlobe is placed on the end of a strip of special paper. The paper contains a chemical that makes it change colour according to the amount of glucose in the blood. Whether the glucose level is low, high or normal can be determined in two ways. The first is, visually, by comparing the end of the strip with a special colour chart on the side of the test strip holder. Types of strips for self blood glucose testing include *Glucostix*, *Dextrostix* and *Visidex*. Instead of comparing the strips to a colour chart, some people use a machine (meter). They insert the strips into the meter and read the correct level of glucose in the blood. The types of meters include: *Dextrochek*, *Glucochek*, *Glucometer* and *Reflolux*.

Blood pressure

The force of the blood on the walls of arteries. Two levels of blood pressure are measured: the higher or *systolic* pressure that occurs each time the heart pushes blood into the vessels, and the lower or *diastolic* pressure that occurs when the heart rests. In a blood-pressure reading of 120/80 mm Hg, for example, 120 mm Hg is the systolic pressure and 80 mm Hg is the diastolic. Such a reading is in the normal range. Too-high blood pressure can cause health problems such as heart attacks and strokes.

Blood vessels

Tubes that act like a system of canals to carry blood – pumped through them by the heart – to and from all parts of the body. The three main types are arteries, veins and capillaries. The blood can carry oxygen and nutrients to the cells and take away waste from them.

Brittle diabetes

A condition in which a person's blood glucose (sugar) level swings quickly from high to low and from low to high, also called 'labile diabetes' or 'unstable diabetes'.

Calorie

A unit of the energy that comes from food. Some foods provide more calories than others. Fats provide many and most vegetables few. Diabetics should follow meal plans with suggested amounts of calories for each meal or snack.

Carbohydrate

One of the three main elements of food. Carbohydrates are mainly sugars and starches, which the body breaks down into glucose, a simple sugar that it uses to feed its cells. The body also uses carbohydrates to make a substance called glycogen, which is stored in the liver and muscles for future use. If the body does not have enough insulin or cannot use the insulin it has, it cannot use carbohydrates for energy as it should. This is diabetes. See: Fat; Protein.

Cholesterol

A fat-like substance found in blood, muscle, liver, brain and other body tissues. The body makes and needs some cholesterol, but too much may cause fat to build up in the arteries and slow down or stop the flow of blood. Butter and egg yolks contain a lot of cholesterol. See: Atherosclerosis.

Coma
A state of unconsciousness that may be due to too-high or too-low a level of glucose (sugar) in the blood. See: Diabetic coma.

Coronary disease
Damage to the heart from too little blood flowing through the vessels feeding the heart muscle because they are blocked with fat or have become thick and hard. This harms the heart muscles. Diabetics are at extra risk of coronary disease.

Diabetic coma
A severe emergency in which a person loses consciousness because the blood glucose (sugar) level is too high and the body has too many ketoacids. The patient usually has a flushed face, dry skin and mouth, rapid and laboured breathing, a fruity breath odour, a rapid and weak pulse and low blood pressure. See: Ketoacidosis.

Diabetic retinopathy
A disease of the small blood vessels of the retina of the eye. At first the tiny vessels grow larger and leak a little fluid into the centre of the retina, blurring the patient's sight ('background retinopathy'). Some 80 per cent of people with this leaking never have serious vision problems, the disease halting at this stage, but a further stage can harm the sight more seriously, when many tiny new blood vessels spread out across the eye. This is called 'neovascularization'. The vessels may break and bleed into the clear gel that fills the centre of the eye, blocking vision, and scar tissue may form near the retina, pulling it away from the back of the eye. This stage, 'proliferative retinopathy', can lead to reduced vision and even blindness.

Diabetologist
A doctor who treats people who have diabetes mellitus.

Dietitian

An expert in nutrition who helps people to plan the kinds and amounts of foods to eat for special health needs. A registered dietitian (SRD) has special therapeutic qualifications.

Endocrinologist

A doctor who treats people who have problems with their endocrine glands. The pancreas is an endocrine gland.

Epidemiology

The study of a disease dealing with how many people have it, where they are, how many new cases arise and how to control it.

Fasting blood glucose test

A method for checking the amount of glucose (sugar) in the blood which can show if a person has diabetes. A blood sample is taken (usually before breakfast, eight hours or so since the last meal eaten). If the blood glucose level is 4 to 6 mmol/L, depending on the type of blood that is tested, it is in the normal range. If the level is over 8 mmol/L it usually indicates diabetes.

Fat

One of the three main classes of foods and a source of energy for the body. Fat helps the body to use some vitamins and helps to keep the skin healthy. It is also the major form in which the body stores energy. In food there are three types of fat: saturated, unsaturated and polyunsaturated.

Saturated fats, which are solid at room temperature, are chiefly animal products such as butter, lard and meat fat. They tend to raise the level of cholesterol in the blood.

Unsaturated (or mono-unsaturated) fats are neutral in that they neither raise nor lower blood cholesterol. Olive oil and peanut oil are examples.

Polyunsaturated fats, which are liquid at room temperature, come from vegetable oils such as corn, cottonseed, sunflower, safflower and soybean. They tend to lower the cholesterol in the blood. See: Carbohydrate; Protein.

Fatty acids
When insulin levels are too low or there is too little glucose (sugar) to use for energy, the body burns fatty acids. The waste products of this process are ketoacids, which raise the acid level in the blood (ketoacidosis), a serious problem. See also: Ketoacidosis.

Fructose
A type of sugar found in many fruits and vegetables and in honey. It is used to sweeten some diet foods.

Gangrene
The death of body tissues, most often caused by a loss of blood flow, especially in the legs and feet.

Glucose
A simple sugar found in the blood. It is the body's main source of energy. It is also called dextrose. See: Blood glucose.

Glycosuria
Glucose (sugar) in the urine.

Glycosylated haemoglobin test
A blood test that measures average blood glucose (sugar) level for the previous two to three months.

Gram
A metric unit of weight. There are 28 grams in an ounce. In some diabetic diet plans the amounts of food are given in grams.

Human insulin (artificial)
An artificial insulin, very like the insulin produced by the body, made in a laboratory using special strains of bacteria called *E. coli*.

Hyperglycaemia
Too much glucose (sugar) in the blood and a sign of diabetes out of control. It occurs when the body has too little insulin or cannot use the insulin it has. Signs are: great thirst and hunger, a dry mouth and a need to urinate often. For those with insulin-dependent diabetes it may lead to diabetic ketoacidosis.

Hyperinsulinism

Too much insulin in the blood. It occurs when the body produces too much insulin on its own or when a patient takes too much, which may make the blood glucose (sugar) level too low. Sufferers feel shaky, nervous, weak, confused and sweaty, and experience headaches and hunger. See: Hypoglycaemia.

Hyperlipidaemia

Too high a level of fats (lipids) in the blood. It occurs when diabetes is out of control.

Hypertension

Blood pressure above the normal range.

Hypoglycaemia

Too little glucose (sugar) in the blood. It occurs when a diabetic has injected too much insulin, eaten too little food or exercised without extra food. A sufferer may feel nervous, shaky, weak and sweaty and experience headaches, blurred vision and hunger. Taking small amounts of sugar, juice or food with sugar usually brings relief within 10–15 minutes.

Insulin

A hormone that helps the body to use glucose (sugar) for energy. It is made by the beta cells of the pancreas, in areas called the islets of Langerhans. When the body cannot produce enough insulin the diabetic must inject it.

Insulin allergy

An allergic or bad reaction to insulin made from pork, beef or bacteria because it is not identical to human insulin or has impurities.

The allergy can be in two forms. When an area of skin becomes red and itchy right round the place where insulin is injected it is called 'local allergy'. When the whole body reacts badly it is called 'systemic allergy'. The patient may have hives or red patches all over the body or may feel changes in the heart rate and the rate of breathing. A doctor may treat the condition by prescribing purified insulin or by desensitization.

Insulin pump

An artificial device that continuously pumps insulin into the body at a low (basal) rate. A plastic tube is attached to the body and a small needle is inserted under the skin. The pump keeps the insulin level steady between meals, and at meal times the patient uses a switch or dial to inject a larger dose (bolus) just before eating. The pump runs on batteries and is used by patients with insulin-dependent diabetes.

Insulin reaction

Too low a level of glucose (sugar) in the blood (hypoglycaemia). It occurs when a diabetic has injected too much insulin, eaten too little food or exercised without extra food. The patient may feel hungry, nauseated, weak, nervous, shaky, confused and sweaty. Taking small amounts of sugar, juice or food with sugar will usually bring relief within 10–15 minutes.

Islet cell transplantation

Moving beta cells from the pancreas of one creature to another. Some day beta cell transplants may help diabetics but it is still in the research stage at present. See: Beta cells.

Islets of Langerhans

Groups of cells in the pancreas which make and secrete hormones that help the body to break down and use food. Named after Paul Langerhans, the German who discovered them in 1869, the cells form clusters comprising five types: beta cells, which make insulin; alpha cells, which make glucagon; delta cells, which make somatostatin; and pancreatic polypeptide cells and D_1 cells, about which little is known.

Ketoacidosis (DKA)

Diabetic ketoacidosis (DKA) occurs when the blood has too little insulin (because of illness, too small an insulin dose or too little exercise) and the body starts using stored fat for its energy, so that ketoacids (ketone bodies) build up in the blood. Ketoacidosis starts slowly and becomes more and more severe, until emergency treatment may be needed. The signs include nausea and vomiting (which can lead to serious loss of water from the body), stomach pain and deep and rapid breathing. If the patient is not given fluids and insulin right away, ketoacidosis can lead to coma and even death.

Ketone bodies

Chemicals that the body produces when there is too little insulin in the blood, and fat is broken down for energy. Ketone bodies can be harmful to body cells. The ketones build up in the blood and 'spill over' into the urine so that the body can get rid of them. The body can also rid itself of one type of ketone, called acetone, through the lungs, which gives the breath a fruity odour. Build-up of ketones for a long time leads to serious illness and coma. See: Ketoacidosis.

Ketonuria

The presence of ketone bodies in the urine, a warning sign of diabetic ketoacidosis.

Ketosis

The build-up of ketone bodies in body tissues and fluids. The signs are nausea, vomiting and stomach pain. Ketosis can lead to ketoacidosis.

Lipid

A term for fat. The body stores fat as energy for future use, like a reserve fuel tank in a car. When the body needs energy it can break the lipids down into fatty acids and burn them like glucose (sugar).

Macrovascular disease

A disease of the large blood vessels that affects long-term diabetics. Fat and blood clots build up in the large blood vessels and stick to their walls.

Meal plan

A guide for controlling the overall intake of calories, carbohydrates, proteins and fats. People with diabetes can use food lists to help them plan a wide range of meals.

Metabolism

The term for how the cells change food chemically so that it can be used to keep the body alive. It is a two-part process. In one, *catabolism*, the body uses food for energy. In the other, *anabolism*, the body uses food to build or mend cells.

Microvascular disease

A disease of the smallest blood vessels that sometimes affects long-term diabetics. The walls of the vessels become so thick and weak that they bleed, leak protein and slow the blood flow through the body, and some cells – notably those in the centre of the eye – may get too little blood and become damaged.

Nonketotic coma

A type of coma induced by too little insulin in the system. A 'nonketotic crisis' means: (1) very high glucose (sugar) levels in the blood; (2) absence of ketoacidosis; (3) great loss of body fluid and (4) a sleepy, confused or comatose state. Nonketotic coma is often the result of some other problem, such as a severe infection or kidney failure.

Non-nutritive/intense sweetener

Used to sweeten foods. Based on saccharin, acesulphame K or aspartame. When in tablet or liquid form adds *NO* calories or carbohydrate. If in powder form it can, because of its combination with a bulking agent, add calories and carbohydrate. Check package carefully before using.

Nutrition

The process by which the body draws nutrients from food and uses them to make or mend its cells.

Nutritionist

A person trained to count the calories and nutrients needed for normal growth and daily activity and to help plan meals and advise on long-term eating habits.

Obesity

The condition of having 20 per cent or more extra body fat than one should for age, height, sex and bone structure. Fat works against the action of insulin and extra body fat is thought to be a risk factor for diabetes.

Oedema

A swelling or puffiness of some part of the body, such as the ankles, caused by water or other body fluids collecting in the cells.

Oral hypoglycaemic agents

Pills or capsules taken to lower the glucose (sugar) level in the blood. They work for some people whose pancreas still makes some insulin, and can help the body in several ways, such as causing the cells in the pancreas to release more insulin or make the body cells more responsive to the insulin produced.

Pancreas

The organ, about the size of a hand and located behind the lower part of the stomach, which produces insulin. It also makes enzymes that help the body to digest food. Throughout the pancreas are the areas called the islets of Langerhans, where groups of cells have special functions. The alpha cells make glucagon, which raises the level of glucose in the blood; the beta cells make insulin and the delta cells make somatostatin. There are also the pancreatic polypeptide cells and the D_1 cells, about which little is known.

Pancreatic transplant

An experimental procedure that involves replacing the pancreas of a diabetic with a healthy pancreas that can make insulin. The healthy pancreas can be from a donor who has just died or from a living relative who can donate half a pancreas and still have enough for his or her own needs.

Peripheral vascular disease (PVD)

Disease in the blood vessels of the arms, legs and feet. Long-term diabetics may get this because their arms, legs and feet are getting too little blood. The signs of PVD are pains in the arms, legs and feet (especially when walking) and foot sores that heal slowly. Though diabetics cannot always avoid PVD, doctors say they have a better chance of doing so if they take good care of their feet, do not smoke and keep their blood pressure and diabetes under good control.

Polydipsia

Abnormal thirst that lasts for long periods. It is a sign of diabetes.

Polyphagia
Abnormal hunger, a sign of diabetes, and often accompanied by loss of weight.

Polyuria
The need to urinate often and in large quantities; a common sign of diabetes.

Postprandial blood glucose
The amount of glucose (sugar) in the blood 1–2 hours after eating.

Protein
One of the three main classes of food. Proteins are made of amino acids, sometimes called the building blocks of the cells. The cells need proteins to grow and to mend themselves. Protein is found in such foods as meat, fish, poultry and eggs. See: Carbohydrates; Fat.

Proteinuria
Too much protein in the urine. This may be a sign of kidney damage.

Risk factor
Anything that increases the chance that a person will get a disease. For example, people are at greater risk of having non-insulin-dependent diabetes if they weigh a lot more (20 per cent or more) than they should.

Saccharin
An artificial sweetener used instead of sugar because it has no calories.

Sorbitol
A sugar alcohol that the body uses slowly. As a sweetener in diet foods it is called a 'nutritive sweetener' because it provides 4 calories per gram, like table sugar and starch.

Sugar
A class of carbohydrates that tastes sweet and is a quick, easy fuel for the body to use. Types of sugar are lactose, glucose, fructose and sucrose.

Sulfonylureas

A group of drugs that lower the glucose (sugar) level in the blood. See: Oral hypoglycaemic agents.

Symptom

A sign of disease, e.g. having to urinate often is a symptom of diabetes.

Triglyceride

A type of blood fat. The body needs insulin to remove this type of fat from the blood. When diabetes is under control and the patient's weight is what it should be, the triglyceride level in the blood is usually about what it should be.

Urine testing

Checking the urine to see if it contains glucose (sugar) or ketones. Special strips of paper or tablets (called reagents) are put into a small amount of urine or urine plus water. Changes in the colour of the strip show the amount of glucose or ketones in the urine.

Some Sources of Additional Help and Information

British Diabetic Association
10 Queen Anne Street
London W1M 0BD
England

The BDA was founded more than 50 years ago to help diabetics. Membership at a yearly fee gives access to free guidance and help on social, welfare and dietetic questions – though not on individual treatment – and a subscription to *Balance*, a bi-monthly newspaper. The Association has over 300 local branches and publishes a variety of patient education materials.

There is also a Diabetes Society in Australia:

Australian Diabetes Society
c/o Dr G. B. Senator, Secretary
Department of Endocrinology
Royal Hobart Hospital
GPO Box 1061 L, Hobart
Tasmania 7001

Pharmaceutical companies that make products for diabetics often have excellent educational materials. Ask your doctor, pharmacist, dietitian or nurse for the names and addresses of companies that provide these.

PART TWO
The recipes

Categories of Food to Help with Meal Planning

Green (go) foods – to use regularly in the diet

Wholewheat (wholemeal) flour and bread
Wholewheat pasta and brown rice
Vegetables – fresh and frozen
Peas, beans and lentils – dried or tinned
Lean red meat, poultry, fish – not fried, nuts
Low- or reduced-fat milk, yogurt, cheese
Reduced-fat spreads
Fresh or frozen fruit, fruit tinned in natural juice
Low-calorie beverages

Amber (caution) foods – to be used with care and not too frequently in the diet

White flour and bread, cornflour and custard powder
Pasta, rice, semolina
Fatty meats, tinned meats
Pâtés and spreads
Full-fat milk, yogurt and cheese
Margarine and butter
Lard, oil, suet dripping
Alcoholic drinks

Red (stop) foods – to be used infrequently as part of a main meal

Glucose, sugar, sweetened cakes, desserts and puddings
Sweets and chocolate, sweetened drinks

Notes on Using
the Recipes

1. If you are unable to obtain all the specific food products called for in a recipe, be sure to make the appropriate adjustments in the nutrient content of the recipe for the items left out.
2. If you are using a sugar substitute in a recipe, follow the specific instructions on the label of the product you select regarding sugar equivalents and specific cooking instructions. These products are different from one another and cannot always be used in the same way. Some sugar substitutes, other than non-nutritive sweeteners, *do* contain calories, and these calories can add up when large amounts are used.
3. Follow directions carefully concerning size of portions served because the nutrient content per serving is based on this size. If a larger or a smaller serving is eaten, make the appropriate adjustments in the nutrient content per serving.
4. Every effort has been made to be as accurate as possible in the nutrient analysis of the recipes and in the specific yields of each recipe but variations will occur because of differences in ingredients and in personal cooking techniques. Therefore, the analysis given is for the whole recipe as well as the *approximate* nutrient content per serving.
5. An asterisk (*) next to the name of a recipe denotes that this dish contains too much salt to be included in the diet of someone on a low-salt diet. You can lower the salt

content of many recipes by using *unsalted* canned tomatoes, tomato purée, stock and soups. You can also reduce the salt content by eliminating salt itself and condiments such as mustard, soy sauce and Worcestershire sauce.

6. NB: Use *either* metric measurements *or* imperial. Do not mix the two.

Appetizers, Soups and Starters

CRAB AND WATER CHESTNUT SPREAD*

175 g/6 oz flaked cooked
  crabmeat (fresh, frozen or
  canned and drained)
200 g/7 oz chopped water
  chestnuts

1 tbsp soy sauce
2 tbsp chopped spring onion
100 g/4 oz reduced-
  calorie mayonnaise

Mix all ingredients. Serve with wholemeal crackers or wholemeal bread.

Total CHO = 40 g
Total Calories = 700
Makes 20 servings each of 2
  tablespoons

1 serving = negligible CHO
  and 35 calories

MAYONNAISE

1 tbsp plus 1½ tsp lemon
  juice
1 tsp Dijon-style mustard
½ tsp salt

1 egg
75 ml/⅛ pint olive oil
150 ml/¼ pint vegetable oil

Measure lemon juice, mustard, salt, egg and one-third oil into blender or food processor. Cover and process for 30 seconds. On high speed, slowly add remaining oil; continue beating until mixture is thick and creamy.

Total CHO = negligible   1 serving = negligible CHO
Total Calories = 2100   and 175 calories
Makes 12 servings each of 2
   tablespoons

EGG MAYONNAISE

---

6 size 3 hard-boiled eggs,   *2 tbsp capers*
   shelled and chilled   *2 tbsp chopped parsley*
8 tbsp of mayonnaise (see
   previous recipe)

Cut eggs lengthwise into halves and place cut side down on a serving platter. Spoon mayonnaise over eggs; garnish with capers and parsley.

Total CHO = negligible   1 serving = negligible CHO
Total Calories = 1200   and 200 calories
Serves 6

FETA CHEESE SPREAD WITH GARLIC AND CHIVES*

225 g/8 oz reduced-fat soft
cheese (e.g. quark-style)
175 g/6 oz feta cheese,
soaked in cold water for 5
minutes then drained
4 anchovy fillets, drained
75 g/3 oz unsalted
margarine, cut into 6
pieces

4 tbsp sour cream
2 cloves garlic, finely
chopped
2 tbsp snipped chives
6 drops red pepper sauce
(Tabasco)
freshly ground white pepper

Place cheeses and anchovy fillets in a blender or food processor. Cover and blend, stopping machine and scraping sides of container with a rubber scraper. Blend in margarine, one piece at a time.

Transfer mixture to a bowl and stir in remaining ingredients. Cover and refrigerate for at least 5 hours. Remove spread 1 hour before serving (if serving as a dip, allow several hours for it to soften).

Total CHO = 10 g
Total Calories = 1360
Makes 16 servings each of 2
tablespoons

1 serving = negligible CHO
and 85 calories

TUNA WITH ALMONDS

1½ envelopes or 3 tsp
  gelatine
150 ml/¼ pint cold water
200 ml/7 fl oz boiling water
450 g/1 lb reduced-fat soft
  cheese (e.g. quark-style)
2 tbsp lemon juice
1 tbsp curry powder
½ tsp salt

¼ tsp garlic powder
5 tbsp finely chopped spring
  onion
50 g/2 oz canned, drained
  pimiento, chopped
2 × 200 g/7 oz cans tuna in
  brine, drained and flaked
150 g/5 oz flaked almonds,
  toasted
parsley and pimiento strips
  to garnish (optional)

Sprinkle gelatine on cold water to soften it. Stir in boiling water until gelatine is dissolved. Beat cheese into gelatine mixture until smooth. Stir in lemon juice, curry powder, salt and garlic powder. Fold in onion, pimiento, tuna and 100 g/4 oz of the almonds. Pour into a 1.1 litre/2 pint mould; chill until firm.

Unmould on to a serving dish. Garnish with remaining almonds and, if desired, parsley and pimiento strips.

Total CHO = 20 g
Total Calories = 1800
Makes 20 servings each of 2
  tablespoons

1 serving = negligible CHO
  and 90 calories

YOGURT DIP

---

225 g/8 oz low-fat natural
   yogurt
⅛ tsp garlic powder
1 heaped tsp prepared
   horseradish

1 tsp mustard
finely chopped dill, tarragon
   or chervil

Mix all ingredients in a small bowl. Cover and refrigerate for several hours.

Total CHO = 15 g
Total Calories = 120
Makes about 8 servings each
   of 2 tablespoons

1 serving = negligible CHO
   and 15 calories

COLD VEGETABLE ANTIPASTO

---

3 tbsp olive oil
450 g/1 lb courgettes, cut
   into 6 mm/¼ in slices
pinch garlic salt
pinch freshly ground pepper

1 small onion, thinly sliced
2 tsp oregano

Heat oven to 180°C/350°F/mark 4. Pour olive oil on a large baking sheet or Swiss roll tin. Add courgette slices and turn with a spatula until coated with oil. Arrange slices so they overlap slightly. Season with garlic, salt and pepper, then sprinkle with onion slices and oregano. Bake for 20 minutes.

Put under a hot grill to brown the top lightly. Cool and serve.

Total CHO = 15 g   1 serving = negligible CHO
Total Calories = 560   and 65 calories
Serves 8

VEGETABLE TEMPURA*

---

vegetable oil for frying   *225 g/8 oz carrots, peeled*
2 egg yolks   *and cut into thin rounds*
275 ml/½ pint ice-cold water *225 g/8 oz cauliflower florets*
50 g/2 oz plain flour   *225 g/8 oz courgettes, cut*
50 g/2 oz wholemeal flour   *into thin rounds*
1 medium green pepper,   *Dipping Sauce (see next*
* seeded and cut into strips*   *recipe)*
* 2.5 cm/1 in wide*
225 g/8 oz broccoli spears,
* trimmed*

Heat oil to 180°C/350°F in a heavy saucepan.

Beat egg yolks; add water and flour and beat until flour is moistened (batter will be lumpy). Dip the prepared vegetables into batter; cook in hot oil until tender and golden brown; about 2 minutes. Drain on paper towels. Serve with Dipping Sauce.

Total CHO = 100 g   Serves 8
Total Calories = 880

Dipping Sauce for Vegetable Tempura*

Mix 150 ml/¼ pint rice wine or dry sherry, 75 ml/⅛ pint soy sauce and 1 tsp finely chopped fresh ginger root.

Total CHO = 15 g
Total Calories = 240
Serves 8 (each serving is negligible CHO and 30 calories)

1 serving of Vegetable Tempura with Dipping Sauce = 15 g CHO and 140 calories

GRILLED STUFFED MUSHROOMS

---

450 g/1 lb small mushrooms
1 medium green pepper, seeded and finely chopped
3 spring onions, chopped
25 g/1 oz margarine
1 large, thin slice wholemeal bread, crumbled
1 tbsp chopped parsley

¼ tsp oregano
pinch cayenne pepper
50 g/2 oz Mozzarella cheese, crumbled
2 tsp dry white wine
50 g/2 oz margarine, melted
paprika

Remove stems from mushrooms and chop; reserve caps for stuffing. Cook and stir mushroom stems, green pepper and onion in the margarine until mushrooms are brown. Stir in breadcrumbs, parsley, oregano, cayenne pepper, cheese and wine, and heat.

Brush mushroom caps with the melted margarine. Heat the grill. Press stuffing into caps and place on grill rack. Sprinkle with paprika and grill until tender; 4 to 5 minutes.

Total CHO = 15 g
Total Calories = 880
Serves 8

1 serving = negligible CHO and 110 calories

CHICKEN WING APPETIZERS

1.4 kg/3 lb chicken wings   *3 cloves garlic, crushed*
150 ml/¼ pint lemon juice   *1 tsp salt*
75 ml/⅛ pint vegetable oil   *1 tsp freshly ground pepper*

Cut bony tips from wings and discard. Separate chicken wings at joint. Place wing halves in a shallow baking dish. Mix lemon juice, oil, garlic, salt and pepper; pour over wing halves. Cover and refrigerate for at least 4 hours, turning occasionally.

Heat oven to 200°C/400°F/mark 6. Remove wing halves from marinade; place on a rack in a roasting tin and bake for 45 minutes.

Wings can be frozen after they are baked. To serve, thaw at room temperature, then grill until hot; 3 to 4 minutes. For a buffet party, allow 7 kg/15 lb to serve 40 people.

Total CHO = negligible   1 serving = negligible CHO
Total Calories = 1280   and 160 calories
Serves 8

MARINATED MUSHROOMS

---

150 g/5 oz quartered   *1 tbsp French mustard*
*   mushrooms*   *1 tbsp chopped parsley*
¼ quantity Vinaigrette
*   Française (see page 120)*

Place mushrooms in a bowl. Mix dressing, mustard and parsley; pour on mushrooms and toss to coat. Serve immediately or marinate for 2 to 3 hours.

Total CHO = negligible
Total Calories = 360
Serves 4

1 serving = negligible CHO
and 90 calories

PORK AND WATERCRESS SOUP*

225 g/8 oz lean pork, very
   finely sliced
1 litre/1¾ pints water
1 litre/1¾ pints chicken
   stock
1 small onion, thinly sliced

1 clove garlic, pressed
¼ tsp pepper
1 tsp salt
1 bunch watercress, cut into
   2.5 cm/1 in pieces

Heat meat and water to boiling in a large saucepan. Reduce heat, cover and simmer for 10 minutes. Add chicken stock, onion, garlic, pepper and salt. Heat to boiling. Reduce heat, cover and simmer for 10 minutes. Stir in watercress; heat to boiling.

Total CHO = negligible
Total Calories = 600
Serves 6

1 serving = negligible CHO
and 100 calories

SPLIT PEA SOUP*

100 g/4 oz dried split peas
1 litre/1¾ pints water
3 tsp instant chicken stock or
   3 chicken stock cubes
1 clove garlic, finely chopped

150 g/5 oz potatoes, peeled
   and sliced
1 medium onion, sliced
1 large carrot, sliced
2 tsp oregano

Place all ingredients in a large saucepan. Heat to boiling, stirring occasionally. Reduce heat, cover and simmer for 1 hour. Pour soup into a blender and blend until smooth. Reheat and serve.

Total CHO = 100 g   1 serving = 15 g CHO and
Total Calories = 500   85 calories
Serves 6

CREAM OF ASPARAGUS SOUP*

450 g/1 lb fresh asparagus,   25 g/1 oz plain flour
   trimmed and cut into 2.5   142 ml/5 fl oz single cream
   cm/1 in pieces   ½ tsp salt
825 ml/1½ pints chicken   ⅛ tsp freshly ground pepper
   stock
50 g/2 oz margarine

Cook asparagus in 275 ml/½ pint of stock until tender; 12 to 15 minutes. Drain and set aside.

Melt margarine in a saucepan. Stir in flour. Cook, stirring constantly, until smooth and bubbly. Stir in remaining stock. Cook, stirring constantly, until mixture thickens and boils. Boil and stir for 1 minute. Stir in cream, seasoning and asparagus, and heat.

Variation
Cream of Broccoli Soup: Substitute 450 g/1 lb broccoli, trimmed and chopped, for the asparagus.

Total CHO = 45 g   1 serving = 10 g CHO and
Total Calories = 840   210 calories
Serves 4

BORSCHT*

1.4 litres/2½ pints chicken stock
175 g/6 oz onion, chopped
175 g/6 oz carrot, peeled and sliced
100 g/4 oz celery stalks, chopped
150 g /5 oz white cabbage, chopped
400 g/14 oz can chopped tomatoes, puréed
1 tbsp salt
1 tbsp white pepper
100 g/4 oz cooked beetroot, finely chopped
non-nutritive sweetener to taste
75 ml/2½ fl oz sour cream

Heat chicken stock, onion, carrot, celery, cabbage, tomato, salt and pepper to boiling in a large saucepan. Reduce heat, cover and simmer for 15 minutes. Stir in beetroot and heat to boiling. Reduce heat and simmer for 5 minutes. Sweeten to taste.

Divide soup among 6 serving bowls; top each with a little of the sour cream.

Total CHO = 60 g
Total Calories = 420
Serves 6

1 serving = 10 g CHO and 70 calories

FARMHOUSE SOUP*

1 litre/1¾ pints water
100 g/4 oz dried haricot
  beans
50 g/2 oz margarine
225 g/8 oz onion, finely
  chopped
1 large leek, finely chopped
1 large stalk celery, finely
  chopped
225 g/8 oz courgettes,
  chopped
350 g/12 oz carrots, peeled
  and chopped

225 g/8 oz potatoes, peeled
  and chopped
800 g/28 oz can whole
  tomatoes
700 ml/1¼ pints chicken
  stock
2 bay leaves
4 sprigs parsley
1 tsp salt
pinch freshly ground pepper
100 g/4 oz brown rice

Heat water to boiling in a medium saucepan. Add beans; heat to boiling and boil for 5 minutes, stirring frequently. Remove from heat and leave beans to soak for 3 to 4 hours.

Melt margarine in a large saucepan. Add onion, leek, celery and half the courgette, carrot and potato. Cook and stir until vegetables are coated; 2 to 3 minutes. Stir in tomatoes, breaking them up with a spoon, stock, bay leaves, parsley, salt and pepper. Heat to boiling. Reduce heat, cover and simmer for 2 hours.

Remove bay leaves and parsley. Stir in remaining courgette, carrot and potato with rice and beans (with liquid). Heat to boiling, stirring occasionally. Reduce heat, cover and simmer for 1 hour.

Total CHO = 225 g   1 serving = 15 g CHO and
Total Calories = 1500   100 calories
Serves 15

COD CHOWDER*

---

425 ml/¾ pint water
350 g/12 oz potatoes, peeled
   and chopped
75 g/3 oz celery, chopped
1 medium onion, chopped
2 tbsp canned pimiento,
   chopped
1½ tsp salt
450 g/1 lb cod, skinned and
   cut into 1 cm/½ in pieces

425 ml/¾ pint skimmed
   milk
1 tbsp wholemeal flour
2 slices lean bacon, grilled
   until crisp and crumbled
1 tbsp margarine
chopped parsley or chives

Heat water, potatoes, celery, onion, pimiento and salt to boiling in a large saucepan. Reduce heat, cover and simmer for 10 minutes. Add fish, cover and simmer until fish and potatoes are tender; about 5 minutes.

Stir in 275 ml/½ pint of the milk. Blend remaining milk and flour; stir into chowder. Heat to boiling, stirring constantly. Stir in bacon and margarine. Sprinkle with chopped parsley or chives.

Total CHO = 90 g
Total Calories = 900
Serves 6

1 serving = 15 g CHO and
   150 calories

GAZPACHO*

---

2 medium tomatoes,
   blanched, skinned and
   chopped
1 medium courgette,
   chopped
1 celery stalk, finely chopped

1 small onion, finely
   chopped
1 clove garlic, crushed
1 litre/1¾ pints
   unsweetened tomato juice
3 lemons

Combine about one-third of the chopped vegetables and one-quarter of the tomato juice in a blender. Blend until vegetables are puréed. Mix puréed vegetables with remaining vegetables in a large bowl. Stir in remaining tomato juice and juice of 2½ lemons. Chill.

Garnish servings with a slice of lemon.

Total CHO = 40 g   1 serving = 10 g CHO and
Total Calories = 160   40 calories
Serves 4

ASPARAGUS VINAIGRETTE

450 g/1 lb fresh asparagus,   *1 tbsp chopped spring onion*
  trimmed   *1½ tsp mustard*
75 ml/⅛ pint vegetable or   *1 clove garlic, crushed*
  olive oil   *¼–½ tsp tarragon*
2 tbsp tarragon vinegar   *⅛ tsp salt*
1 tbsp lemon juice

Cook asparagus, covered, in a large frying pan in 2.5 cm/1 in of salted water (½ tsp salt to 275 ml/½ pint water) just until crisp-tender; 5 to 10 minutes. Drain and place asparagus in a shallow dish. Mix remaining ingredients; pour over asparagus. Cover and refrigerate for 2 hours.

Drain before serving. (Marinade may be used as salad dressing.)

Total CHO = 20 g   1 serving = 5 g CHO and 60
Total Calories = 240   calories
Serves 4

VEGETABLE AND BARLEY SOUP

1 tbsp vegetable oil
225 g/8 oz onion, chopped
150 g/5 oz celery, thinly
  sliced
225 g/8 oz carrot, thinly
  sliced
1 clove garlic, finely chopped
1.4 litres/2½ pints beef stock
400 g/14 oz can tomatoes

2 tbsp Worcestershire sauce
1 bay leaf
1–1½ tsp salt
½ tsp basil
225 g/8 oz French beans, cut
  into 4 cm/1½ in pieces (or
  use 275 g/10 oz frozen cut
  French beans)
150 g/5 oz pot barley
freshly ground pepper

Heat oil in a 4–5 litre/8 pint saucepan or kettle. Add onion, celery, carrot and garlic; cook and stir over medium heat for 2 minutes. Add remaining ingredients; heat to boiling. Reduce heat, cover and simmer until barley is tender; 1 to 1½ hours. *Note:* If using frozen beans, do not add until the last 10 minutes of cooking.

Total CHO = 180 g
Total Calories = 900
Serves 12

1 serving = 15 g CHO and
  75 calories

BEEF KEBABS

---

450 g/1 lb lean minced beef
1 medium slice wholemeal
    bread, soaked in water
    and squeezed
2 medium onions, finely
    chopped
2 cloves garlic, crushed
2 tsp chopped fresh
    coriander or ½ tsp ground
    coriander

¼ tsp cayenne pepper
2 tsp curry powder
½ tsp salt
2.5 cm/1 in piece fresh
    ginger root, chopped
1 or 2 green chilli peppers,
    thinly sliced
¼ tsp cloves
½ tsp cinnamon
3 tbsp vegetable oil

Mix all ingredients except oil. Shape mixture into 50 small balls. Heat oil in a large frying pan. Cook meatballs in oil until done and brown. Serve as appetizers. (Mixture can be shaped into larger meatballs for a main dish.)

Total CHO = 20 g
Total Calories = 1300
Serves 10

1 serving of 5 meatballs =
    negligible CHO and 130
    calories

Salads and Salad Dressings

CURRIED MIXED FRUIT SALAD

Select 450 g/1 lb of prepared fruit, e.g. equal quantities of pineapple chunks or slices, seedless green grapes, apple slices, banana slices and melon wedges. Arrange on a plate. Serve with Curried Fruit Salad Dressing (below).

Curried Fruit Salad Dressing

175 ml/6 fl oz low-fat
   natural yogurt
4 tbsp reduced-calorie
   mayonnaise
non-nutritive intense
   sweetener to taste

1 tsp curry powder
⅛ tsp salt
1 tsp finely chopped fresh
   ginger root
1 tsp lemon juice

Mix all ingredients. Cover and refrigerate for at least 3 hours.

Total CHO = 60 g
Total Calories = 420
Serves 6

1 serving of fruit and
   dressing = about 10 g
   CHO and 70 calories

TOMATOES WITH MOZZARELLA

---

675 g/1½ lb tomatoes,
   thinly sliced
225 g/8 oz Mozzarella
   cheese, sliced

1 tbsp olive oil
chopped fresh basil or chives
freshly ground pepper

Arrange slices of tomato and cheese alternately on salad plates. Sprinkle olive oil on top and garnish with basil or chives. Season with pepper.

Total CHO = 20 g
Total Calories = 880
Serves 4

1 serving = 5 g CHO and
   220 calories

SUMMIT SALAD

---

100 g/4 oz chicory, thinly
   sliced
1 small lettuce, torn into
   bite-size pieces
1 small bunch watercress,
   trimmed
2 large oranges, peeled and
   chopped

½ medium green pepper,
   seeded and cut into thin
   strips 2.5 cm/1 in long
1 small (150 g/5 oz) avocado
   pear, peeled, stoned and
   chopped

Toss all ingredients except dressing in a large bowl. Tarragon Salad Dressing (page 119) is a good dressing for this salad.

Total CHO = 20 g
Total Calories = 360
Serves 6

1 serving = negligible CHO
   and 60 calories

LENTIL SALAD

---

225 g/8 oz whole lentils,
  cooked until tender but
  still firm
1 medium onion, chopped
2 celery stalks, diced
275 g/10 oz courgettes,
  chopped
1 tsp dry mustard
¼ tsp garlic powder or 1
  clove garlic, finely
  chopped

2 tsp oregano
¼ tsp freshly ground pepper
2 tbsp wine vinegar
3 tbsp vegetable oil
4 small firm tomatoes,
  quartered
100 g/4 oz Mozzarella
  cheese, finely chopped or
  grated
lettuce leaves to serve

Combine all ingredients except tomatoes and cheese in a large bowl. Toss until lentils and vegetables are coated with oil. Cover and refrigerate for several hours to blend flavours.

Mix in tomato quarters and cheese; serve on lettuce leaves.

Total CHO = 140 g
Total Calories = 1505
Serves 7

1 serving = 20 g CHO and
  215 calories

WHITE KIDNEY BEAN AND TUNA SALAD

---

200 g/7 oz can tuna in brine,
  drained and flaked
440 g/15½ oz can white
  kidney beans, drained
4 tbsp vegetable oil
1 tbsp lemon juice
¼ tsp freshly ground pepper
¼ tsp salt

1 clove garlic, finely chopped
1 medium onion, chopped
lettuce leaves
½ medium green pepper,
  seeded and cut into rings
1 large tomato, cut into
  wedges
3 tbsp chopped parsley

Combine tuna, beans, oil, lemon juice, pepper, salt, garlic and onion in a bowl; toss until ingredients are coated with oil. Cover and refrigerate for at least 1 hour.

Serve on lettuce leaves and garnish with green pepper rings, tomato wedges and parsley.

Total CHO = 60 g   1 serving = 10 g CHO and
Total Calories = 1100   185 calories
Serves 6 (small servings)

CRISPY GREEN SALAD

1 very large cos lettuce or 2
   small ones
1 tbsp chopped spring onion
50 g/2 oz Emmental cheese,
   diced
1 tbsp red wine vinegar

⅛ tsp garlic powder
¼ tsp dry mustard
⅛ tsp salt
pinch freshly ground pepper
3 tbsp olive or vegetable oil

Tear lettuce into bite-sized pieces and place in a salad bowl. Add onion and cheese. Shake remaining ingredients in a screw-top jar; pour over ingredients in bowl and toss.

Total CHO = negligible   1 serving = negligible CHO
Total Calories = 640   and 80 calories
Serves 8

SALAD COMBO

---

1 small bunch watercress
100 g/4 oz chicory, sliced
75 g/3 oz courgettes, thinly
   sliced
2 medium tomatoes, sliced

1 small round lettuce,
   shredded
4–5 spring onions, thinly
   sliced
50 g/2 oz curly endive,
   shredded

Mix all ingredients together in a large salad bowl.

Total CHO = negligible
Total Calories = 75
Serves 5

1 serving = negligible CHO
   and 15 calories

CRAB SALAD

---

100 g/4 oz cooked crabmeat
675 g/1½ lb asparagus
   spears, cooked, drained
   and chilled
6 large lettuce leaves

Lemon-caper Dressing (see
   below)
paprika
3 tomatoes, cut into wedges

Flake crabmeat; remove any shell particles or cartilage. Place asparagus spears on lettuce leaves. Top with crabmeat and about 2 tbsp of dressing. Sprinkle with paprika and garnish with tomato wedges.

Total CHO = 10 g
Total Calories = 210
Serves 6

1 serving = negligible CHO
   and 35 calories

Lemon-caper Dressing

---

100 g/4 oz reduced-calorie
 mayonnaise
1 tbsp drained capers
½ tsp dry mustard

½ tsp Worcestershire sauce
2 drops red pepper sauce
 (Tabasco)

Mix all the ingredients together.

Total CHO = negligible
Total Calories = 360
Serves 6

1 serving = negligible CHO
 and 60 calories

HEALTH SALAD

½ quantity Vinaigrette
 Française (page 120)
1 tbsp Dijon mustard
100 g/4 oz Mozzarella
 cheese, finely diced
1 medium green pepper,
 seeded and finely diced

1 medium courgette, sliced
6 radishes, quartered
8 cup mushrooms, quartered
6 spring onions, chopped
3 tomatoes, cut into chunks

Mix dressing and mustard in a salad bowl. Add remaining
ingredients and toss. Cover and refrigerate for 1 hour.

Total CHO = 10 g
Total Calories = 1000
Serves 5

1 serving = negligible CHO
 and 200 calories

CAESAR SALAD*

---

1 clove garlic, halved
75 ml/⅛ pint olive oil
1 tsp Worcestershire sauce
½ tsp salt
¼ tsp dry mustard
freshly ground pepper
1 large cos lettuce or 2 small
   ones, washed and chilled

1 size 3 egg, very lightly
   boiled and cooled in cold
   water
1 lemon
25 g/1 oz grated Parmesan
   cheese

Just before serving rub a large salad bowl with the clove of garlic. A few small pieces can be left in the bowl. Add oil, Worcestershire sauce, salt, mustard and pepper; mix thoroughly.

Tear lettuce into bite-sized pieces over the bowl. Toss until leaves glisten. Break egg on top and squeeze lemon juice over. Toss until leaves are well coated. Sprinkle cheese over salad and toss again.

Total CHO = negligible
Total calories = 780
Serves 6

1 serving = negligible CHO
   and 130 calories

Note: Caesar Salad traditionally includes garlic croûtons. If these are included allow 15 g CHO and 100 calories for every medium slice of bread lightly spread with butter or margarine.

COURGETTE SALAD

---

225 g/8 oz spinach
175 g/6 oz small firm
    tomatoes, quartered

1 medium courgette, thinly
    sliced
3 spring onions, thinly sliced

Wash spinach; remove stems and tear leaves into bite-sized pieces. Dry and chill.

    Combine spinach, tomatoes, courgette and onion in a salad bowl and toss.

Total CHO = 20 g
Total Calories = 120
Serves 6

1 serving = negligible CHO
    and 20 calories

Note: This can be served with ¼ quantity Spicy Italian Salad Dressing (page 118).

SPINACH SALAD

---

275 g/10 oz spinach
1 tsp grated onion
¼ tsp salt
pinch freshly ground pepper
1 tsp Dijon mustard

1 tbsp red wine vinegar
1 tbsp olive oil
lemon juice
5 radishes, thinly sliced

Wash spinach; remove stems and tear leaves into bite-sized pieces. Dry and chill.

    Beat onion, salt, pepper, mustard, vinegar and oil with a fork. Stir in lemon juice to taste (if dressing separates, beat again). Pour dressing over spinach in a salad bowl; add radish slices and toss.

Total CHO = 10 g
Total Calories = 240
Serves 6

1 serving = negligible CHO
and 40 calories

BROWN RICE AND CUCUMBER SALAD

150 g/5 oz brown rice,
  cooked and cooled
100 g/4 oz mushrooms,
  sliced
2–3 spring onions, chopped
1 medium (175 g/6 oz)
  cucumber, seeded and
  diced
1 stalk celery, chopped

1 tomato, chopped
225 g/8 oz frozen peas,
  thawed and lightly cooked
1 tbsp chopped parsley
½ quantity Oil-and-vinegar
  Dressing (page 120)

Combine rice, mushrooms, onion, cucumber, celery, tomato, peas and parsley in a large bowl. Toss with enough dressing to coat ingredients. Cover and refrigerate for at least 2 hours.

Total CHO = 120 g
Total Calories = 1040
Serves 8

1 serving = 15 g CHO and
130 calories

Note: If wishing to reduce calories and fat serve the dressing separately. Salad without dressing = 15 g CHO and 90 calories per serving.

SWEET-AND-SOUR FRUIT SLAW

---

1 small white cabbage
(about 350 g/12 oz),
coarsely shredded
1 medium apple, cored and
chopped
150 g/5 oz green or black
grapes, halved and seeded
312 g/11 oz can mandarin
orange sections in natural
juice, drained

25 g/1 oz raisins
225 g/8 oz carton low-fat
cottage cheese
4 tbsp skimmed milk
3 tbsp lemon juice
2 tbsp salad oil

Combine cabbage, apple, grapes, orange sections and raisins. Put the cheese, milk, lemon juice and oil into a blender and process until smooth. Pour dressing over cabbage mixture and toss. Chill before serving.

Total CHO = 100 g
Total Calories = 900
Serves 10

1 serving = 10 g CHO and
90 calories

LEMONY FRENCH DRESSING

---

75 ml/⅛ pint vegetable oil
2 tbsp vinegar
2 tbsp lemon juice
½ tsp salt

¼ tsp dry mustard
¼ tsp paprika
non-nutritive intense
sweetener to taste

Shake all ingredients in a screw-top jar. Refrigerate for at least 1 hour. Shake before serving.

Total CHO = negligible
Total Calories = 700
Serves 4–6

1 serving = negligible CHO
and about 115–175
calories

HERBED MAYONNAISE

---

225 g/8 oz reduced-calorie
   mayonnaise
2 tsp lemon juice
1 tbsp chopped parsley

1 tbsp chopped chives
½ tsp tarragon
½ tsp chervil

Mix all ingredients in a small bowl. Cover and refrigerate for
1 to 2 hours. Serve with fish.

Total CHO = negligible
Total Calories = 360
Serves 8

1 serving = negligible CHO
and 45 calories

HERB SALAD DRESSING

---

200 ml/7 fl oz vegetable oil
75 ml/⅛ pint white wine
   vinegar
1 spring onion, finely
   chopped

1 tbsp chopped parsley or 1
   tsp parsley flakes
1 tsp dry mustard
1 tsp thyme
1 tsp tarragon
1 clove garlic, split

Shake all ingredients in a screw-top jar. Refrigerate for at
least 4 hours. Remove garlic clove before using.

Total CHO = negligible
Total Calories = 1800
Serves 10

1 serving = negligible CHO
and 180 calories

SPICY ITALIAN SALAD DRESSING

---

200 ml/7 fl oz vegetable oil
75 ml/⅛ pint red wine
  vinegar
⅛ tsp crushed dried red
  pepper
1 clove garlic, split
¼ tsp garlic powder
2 tsp dry mustard

1 tbsp very finely chopped
  onion
¼ tsp salt
3 peppercorns
¾ tsp oregano
½ tsp basil
¼ tsp marjoram
3 or 4 drops red pepper sauce
  (Tabasco)

Shake all ingredients in a screw-top jar. Refrigerate for at least 4 hours. Remove garlic clove and peppercorns and shake before using.

Total CHO = negligible
Total Calories = 1800
Serves 10

1 serving = negligible CHO
  and 180 calories

ITALIAN SALAD DRESSING

---

175 ml/6 fl oz vegetable oil
4 tbsp red wine vinegar
⅛ tsp salt
⅛ tsp freshly ground pepper
½ tsp dry mustard

¼ tsp paprika
⅛ tsp cayenne pepper
½ tsp oregano
½ tsp marjoram
1 clove garlic, split
¼ tsp basil

Shake all ingredients in a screw-top jar. Refrigerate for at least 4 hours. Remove garlic and shake before using.

Total CHO = negligible
Total Calories = 1600
Serves 8

1 serving = negligible CHO
and 200 calories

TARRAGON SALAD DRESSING

175 ml/6 fl oz vegetable oil
4 tbsp tarragon white wine
   vinegar
1 tsp chopped parsley
½ tsp tarragon, crushed
1 clove garlic, split

⅛ tsp salt
1 tsp dry mustard
2 tsp very finely chopped
   onion
pinch freshly ground pepper

Shake all ingredients in a screw-top jar. Refrigerate for at least 4 hours. Remove garlic and shake before using.

Total CHO = negligible
Total Calories = 1600
Serves 8

1 serving = negligible CHO
and 200 calories

LEMON DRESSING

4 tbsp vegetable oil
2 tbsp lemon juice
1 tbsp plus 1½ tsp tarragon
   vinegar

1 tsp chopped parsley
¼ tsp freshly ground pepper

Shake all ingredients in a screw-top jar.

Total CHO = negligible
Total Calories = 540
Serves 6

1 serving = negligible CHO
and 90 calories

VINAIGRETTE FRANÇAISE*

---

4 tbsp wine vinegar
150 ml/¼ pint vegetable oil
1 tsp salt
pinch freshly ground pepper

1 clove garlic, split
1 tsp dry salad herbs
1 tsp dry mustard

Shake all ingredients in a screw-top jar. Refrigerate for at least 1 hour. Remove garlic and shake before using.

Total CHO = negligible
Total Calories = 1360
Makes 8 servings each of 2
   tablespoons

1 serving = negligible CHO
   and 170 calories

OIL-AND-VINEGAR DRESSING

---

2 tbsp red wine vinegar
75 ml/⅛ pint olive oil
½ tsp salt
2 drops red pepper sauce
   (Tabasco)

¼ tsp freshly ground pepper
⅛ tsp dry mustard

Measure all ingredients into a screw-top jar. Cover and shake.

Total CHO = negligible
Total Calories = 690
Makes 6 servings each of 1
   tablespoon

1 serving = negligible CHO
   and 115 calories

ZERO SALAD DRESSING

---

1 tsp or ½ envelope gelatine
275 ml/½ pint unsalted
    tomato juice

2 tbsp vinegar
1 clove garlic, split
¼ tsp red pepper sauce
1 tbsp vegetable oil

Sprinkle gelatine on 3 tbsp of the tomato juice in a small saucepan to soften it. Stir over low heat until gelatine is dissolved; 2 to 3 minutes. Remove from heat; stir in remaining ingredients. Cover and refrigerate. Remove garlic and shake or stir before using.

Total CHO = 10 g
Total Calories = 200
Serves 10

1 serving = negligible CHO
    and 20 calories

FRENCH DRESSING

---

75 ml/⅛ pint vegetable oil
3 tbsp wine vinegar
2 tbsp lemon juice
1 tbsp finely chopped onion
    or chives

2 tsp chopped parsley
1¾ tsp paprika
½ tsp basil
⅛ tsp pepper
1½ cloves garlic, split

Shake all ingredients in a screw-top jar. Refrigerate for at least 12 hours to blend flavours. Remove garlic and shake before using.

Total CHO = negligible
Total Calories = 660
Serves 6

1 serving = negligible CHO
    and 110 calories

ZESTY FRENCH DRESSING

---

150 ml/¼ pint vegetable oil *1 tsp paprika*
6 tbsp lemon juice or vinegar *1 tsp dry mustard*
1 tsp red pepper sauce *non-nutritive intense*
  (Tabasco)   *sweetener to taste*
      (optional)

Shake all ingredients in a screw-top jar. Refrigerate.

Total CHO = negligible 1 serving = negligible CHO
Total Calories = 1360   and 170 calories
Serves 8

SLIMMERS' MAYONNAISE

---

450 g/1 lb low-fat cottage *1 tbsp lemon juice*
  cheese, sieved   *2 tbsp olive oil*
4 tbsp low-fat natural *1 tbsp white pepper*
  yogurt   *dash red pepper sauce*
1 egg   *(Tabasco)*
1–2 tsp dry mustard

Measure the cheese, yogurt and egg into a blender. Process until smooth. Add remaining ingredients and mix until smooth. Refrigerate. This mayonnaise will keep for 5 days in refrigerator.

Total CHO = 10 g 1 serving = negligible CHO
Total Calories = 800   and 40 calories
Serves 20

Vegetables

SAUTÉED CUCUMBERS*

---

2 × 350 g/12 oz cucumbers   *¼ tsp pepper*
50 g/2 oz margarine   *dash red pepper sauce*
1 tsp salt   *(Tabasco)*

Cut cucumbers into 6 mm/¼ in slices. Melt margarine in a large frying pan. Add cucumber slices, salt, pepper and pepper sauce. Cook and stir until cucumbers are crisp-tender. Drain well.

Total CHO = 10 g   1 serving = negligible CHO
Total Calories = 400   and 100 calories
Serves 4

BRAISED CELERY

---

550 ml/1 pint chicken stock   *2 celery hearts, quartered*

Heat stock to boiling. Add celery and cover. Reduce heat and simmer until celery is tender; about 20 minutes.

Total CHO = negligible   1 serving = negligible CHO
Total Calories = 60   and 15 calories
Serves 4

TURNIP PURÉE

---

675 g/1½ lb turnips, peeled
and cubed
3 tbsp skimmed milk

1 tbsp margarine
⅛ tsp nutmeg
salt and white pepper

Heat 2.5 cm/1 in salted water in a saucepan (½ tsp salt to 275 ml/½ pint water) to boiling. Add turnips; cover and heat to boiling. Reduce heat and cook until tender; 15 to 20 minutes. Drain and mash turnips. Add milk, margarine and nutmeg and beat until smooth. Season with salt and white pepper.

Total CHO = 20 g
Total Calories = 240
Serves 4

1 serving = 5 g CHO and 60
calories

WINTER VEGETABLE PLATTER

---

175 g/6 oz cabbage,
shredded
150 g/5 oz turnip, peeled and
diced
150 g/5 oz parsnip, diced
150 g/5 oz sweet potato,
peeled and diced

150 g/5 oz carrot, peeled and
diced
50 g/2 oz margarine
1 tbsp chopped parsley
1 tbsp dill weed
pinch each salt and pepper

Layer vegetables in order listed in a steamer. Steam until tender; 15 to 20 minutes. Arrange vegetables on a warm serving dish. Melt margarine in a small frying pan, stir in parsley and dill weed. Season with salt and pepper and pour over vegetables.

Total CHO = 60 g   1 serving = 10 g CHO and
Total Calories = 660   110 calories
Serves 6

RED AND GREEN STIR-FRY

450 g/1 lb courgettes   1 tbsp margarine
1 medium red pepper   salt and freshly ground
1 large onion   pepper
1 tbsp olive oil

Cut courgettes into 7 cm/3 in long narrow strips. Cut red pepper into 5 cm/2 in long narrow strips, discarding seeds. Cut onion into thin slices and separate into rings.

Heat oil and margarine in a large frying pan. Add vegetables, cook and stir until tender; about 5 minutes. Season with salt and pepper.

Total CHO = 20 g   1 serving = 5 g CHO and 95
Total Calories = 380   calories
Serves 4

VEGETABLE PLATTER*

1 medium head of celery   450 g/1 lb broccoli florets
1 medium cauliflower (about   (fresh or frozen)
   900 g/2 lb)   1 tbsp margarine
700 ml/1¼ pints beef stock   25 g/1 oz toasted sesame
¾ tsp salt   seed
450 g/1 lb carrot, peeled and   2 tbsp snipped chives
   sliced   2 tbsp lemon juice

Cut off root end of celery and remove coarse outer ribs. Wash celery. Cut the bunch crosswise once so bottom section is 13 cm/5 in long (refrigerate top section for later use). Cut bottom section crosswise into 4 equal pieces and tie each one into a bundle with string.

Remove outer leaves and stalk of cauliflower. Cut off any discoloration on florets; wash cauliflower thoroughly. Heat beef stock and salt to boiling in a 3.4 litre/6 pint saucepan. Add cauliflower and heat to boiling. Reduce heat, cover and simmer for 10 minutes. Place celery bundles under cauliflower. Cover and simmer until cauliflower is tender; 15 to 20 minutes.

Heat 2.5 cm/1 in salted water to boiling. Add carrot slices, return to the boil, cover and simmer until crisp-tender; 12 to 15 minutes. Drain.

Heat 1 cm/½ in salted water to boiling. Place broccoli florets in steam basket. Steam for 10 minutes until crisp-tender. Remove from basket.

Heat margarine in a small saucepan. Cook and stir sesame seed, chives and lemon juice until heated through; about 5 minutes.

Place cauliflower in centre of a large serving dish. Arrange carrot slices, broccoli and celery around it. Pour the lemon and sesame seed sauce over.

Total CHO = 60 g   1 serving = 10 g CHO and
Total Calories = 600   100 calories
Serves 6

BROCCOLI WITH GARLIC

900 g/2 lb broccoli   150 ml/¼ pint beef stock
2 tbsp olive oil   1 lemon, thinly sliced
3 cloves garlic, crushed

Remove tough ends from lower stems of the broccoli. Wash and divide into clusters. If stems are thicker than 2.5 cm/1 in across, make lengthways gashes in each stem.

Heat a wok or large frying pan over high heat for 30 seconds. Add oil and heat for another 30 seconds. Rotate pan to coat with oil. Add garlic; stir until brown. Remove garlic; reduce heat to medium. Add broccoli and cook, stirring occasionally, until it is bright green; 3 to 4 minutes. Add beef stock, cover and simmer for 3 to 4 minutes. Remove broccoli and garnish with lemon slices.

Total CHO = 20 g   1 serving = negligible CHO
Total Calories = 420   and 70 calories
Serves 6

BROCCOLI AND CARROTS*

2 tbsp olive oil   4 tbsp beef stock
350 g/12 oz broccoli, broken   4 tbsp soy sauce
   into florets   salt and freshly ground
450 g/1 lb carrots, peeled   pepper
   and diagonally sliced

Heat a wok or large frying pan over high heat for 30 seconds. Add oil to pan and heat for another 30 seconds. Rotate pan to coat with oil. Reduce heat; add broccoli and carrots. Cook and stir vegetables until broccoli is bright green. Stir in stock and soy sauce; cover and cook for 1 to 2 minutes. Season with salt and pepper.

Total CHO = 30 g   1 serving = 5 g CHO and 70
Total Calories = 420   calories
Serves 6

BROCCOLI CASSEROLE*

---

275 g/10 oz frozen broccoli
    florets
275 g/10 oz can cream of
    mushroom soup
50 g/2 oz mature Cheddar
    cheese, grated
1 small onion, finely
    chopped
50 g/2 oz reduced-calorie
    mayonnaise

½ tsp dry mustard
1 egg, beaten
salt and freshly ground
    pepper
4 wholemeal crackers,
    crumbled
4 tbsp bran

Heat oven to 180°C/350°F/mark 4. Cook broccoli as directed on packet, but decrease cooking time by 5 minutes. Turn broccoli into a large bowl. Stir in soup, cheese, onion, mayonnaise, mustard and egg. Season with salt and pepper. Pour into an oiled 1.1 litre/2 pint casserole. Mix cracker crumbs and bran; sprinkle over top. Bake for 45 minutes until golden brown.

Total CHO = 40 g
Total Calories = 800
Serves 4

1 serving = 10 g CHO and
    200 calories

AUBERGINE PROVENÇALE

---

450 g/1 lb tomatoes,
    blanched, skinned, seeded
    and chopped
2 small cloves garlic, crushed
4 tbsp olive oil

salt and freshly ground
    pepper
1 large aubergine (450 g/1
    lb), cut into 2 cm/¾ in
    cubes
chopped parsley

Cook and stir tomatoes and garlic in 1 tbsp oil until tomatoes are tender; about 4 minutes. Season with salt and pepper. Remove from heat and keep warm.

Heat 3 tbsp oil in a large frying pan over medium heat. Add aubergine; cook and stir until it is tender; 5 to 10 minutes. Stir in tomato mixture and cook for 3 minutes longer. Garnish with parsley.

Total CHO = 20 g   1 serving = negligible CHO
Total Calories = 660   and 110 calories
Serves 6

STEAMED SUMMER VEGETABLES

---

450 g/1 lb courgettes, sliced   2 tbsp margarine
225 g/8 oz carrots, peeled   2 tbsp finely chopped spring
    and sliced   onion
salt and freshly ground   2 tbsp finely chopped tomato
    pepper

Heat 1 cm/½ in water in a saucepan to boiling. Place steamer basket with courgette and carrot slices over saucepan. Cover and steam until carrots are crisp-tender; 10 minutes.

Turn vegetables into a warm serving dish; season with salt and pepper. Add margarine and turn until vegetables are coated. Sprinkle onion and tomato on top.

Total CHO = 30 g   1 serving = 5 g CHO and 65
Total Calories = 390   calories
Serves 6

CAULIFLOWER WITH CHEESE AND BACON

1 medium cauliflower (about
  900 g/2 lb)
100 g/4 oz Cheddar cheese,
  grated

50 g/2 oz lean back bacon,
  grilled until crisp and
  crumbled

Remove outer leaves and stalk of cauliflower. Cut off any discoloration on florets. Wash cauliflower and leave whole. Heat 1 cm/½ in water in a large saucepan to boiling. Place steamer basket with cauliflower over saucepan. Cover and steam until tender; 30 to 40 minutes. Place cauliflower in a warm serving dish; sprinkle cheese and bacon on top.

Total CHO = 10 g
Total Calories = 540
Serves 6

1 serving = negligible CHO
  and 90 calories

SPINACH WITH TOMATOES

450 g/1 lb spinach
2 cloves garlic, crushed
2 tbsp olive oil

400 g/14 oz can tomatoes,
  drained and chopped
salt and freshly ground
  pepper

Place spinach in a saucepan with just the water which clings to leaves. Cover and cook for about 3 minutes. Chop and drain thoroughly.

Cook and stir garlic in oil over medium heat for 1 to 2 minutes (do not overcook). Stir in tomatoes; season with salt and pepper. Reduce heat and simmer for 2 to 3 minutes. Stir in spinach and simmer until hot; about 10 minutes.

Total CHO = 20 g
Total Calories = 400
Serves 4

1 serving = 5 g CHO and
100 calories

STIR-FRIED COURGETTES

*50 g/2 oz lean back
   bacon*
4 tbsp olive oil
*1 bunch spring onions, finely
   sliced*

*450 g/1 lb courgettes, cut
   into 8 cm/3 in narrow
   strips*
*25 g/1 oz grated Parmesan
   cheese*

Grill bacon until crisp and cut into small pieces.

Heat oil in a wok or frying pan until hot. Rotate pan to coat with oil. Add spring onions; stir-fry until tender. (Do not brown.) Add courgette and bacon; cook and stir over medium heat until courgette is crisp-tender, 3 to 4 minutes. Stir in cheese.

Total CHO = 15 g
Total Calories = 800
Serves 4

1 serving = negligible CHO
and 200 calories

CARROTS WITH WATER CHESTNUTS
AND ORANGE SECTIONS

*450 g/1 lb carrots, peeled
   and cut into 8 cm/3 in
   narrow strips*
*salt and freshly ground
   pepper*
2 tbsp margarine

*275 g/10 oz can whole water
   chestnuts, drained and
   sliced into halves*
*3 large oranges, peeled,
   sectioned and cut up*

Heat 1 cm/½ in water in a saucepan to boiling. Place steamer basket with carrots over pan, cover and steam until carrots are crisp-tender; 10 to 15 minutes. Turn carrots into a warm bowl; season with salt and pepper. Add margarine, water chestnuts and orange pieces and toss.

Total CHO = 80 g   1 serving = 20 g CHO and
Total Calories = 560   140 calories
Serves 4

STEAMED CARROTS WITH DILL WEED

450 g/1 lb carrots, peeled   *1 tsp dry mustard*
  and sliced   *1 tsp dill weed*
2 tbsp margarine
pinch freshly ground pepper

Heat 1 cm/½ in water in a saucepan to boiling. Place steamer basket with carrots over saucepan. Cover and steam until carrots are crisp-tender; 10 to 12 minutes.

Melt margarine; mix in pepper, mustard and dill weed. Pour over carrots and toss.

Total CHO = 20 g   1 serving = 5 g CHO and 80
Total Calories = 320   calories
Serves 4

RATATOUILLE*

---

900 g/2 lb aubergines, peeled
   and cut into 2.5 cm/1 in
   cubes
450 g/1 lb courgettes, cut
   into quarters and sliced 2
   cm/¾ in thick
1 large Spanish onion, cut
   into quarters and sliced 2
   cm/¾ in thick

2 tbsp olive oil
400 g/14 oz can chopped
   tomatoes
50 g/2 oz hard cheese, grated

Cook and stir aubergine, courgette and onion in oil in a large saucepan over medium heat for 10 minutes. Stir in tomatoes; heat to boiling. Reduce heat, cover and simmer for 30 minutes, stirring occasionally, until vegetables are tender. Sprinkle cheese on top.

Total CHO = 60 g
Total Calories = 780
Serves 6

1 serving = 10 g CHO and
   130 calories

GREEN BEANS MILANO

---

1 medium onion, finely
   chopped
1 clove garlic, finely chopped
2 tbsp vegetable oil
225 g/8 oz tomatoes,
   blanched, skinned and
   coarsely chopped

675 g/1½ lb runner beans,
   trimmed and sliced
75 ml/⅛ pint water
¼ tsp salt
½ tsp pepper
½ tsp oregano

Cook and stir onion and garlic in oil in a large saucepan until onion is tender; 3 to 4 minutes. Add remaining ingredients;

heat to boiling. Reduce heat, cover and simmer until beans are crisp-tender; about 30 minutes.

Total CHO = 30 g
Total Calories = 480
Serves 6

1 serving = 5 g CHO and 80 calories

PETITS POIS*

---

1 small lettuce, shredded
450 g/1 lb frozen petits pois
4 sprigs parsley, tied
   together
½ tsp salt

1 tsp thyme
25 g/1 oz margarine
2 tbsp water
1 tbsp finely chopped onion

Place lettuce in a saucepan. Add remaining ingredients. Heat to boiling, stirring once or twice. Reduce heat, cover and simmer for 10 minutes. Remove parsley sprigs before serving.

Total CHO = 40 g
Total Calories = 460
Serves 4

1 serving = 10 g CHO and 115 calories

BROWN RICE PILAF*

---

1 medium onion, chopped
1 medium green pepper,
   seeded and diced
1 medium red pepper, seeded
   and diced
1 tbsp vegetable oil

75 g/3 oz mushrooms,
   chopped
200 g/7 oz brown rice
425 ml/¾ pint chicken stock

Cook and stir onion and green and red peppers in oil in a large saucepan over medium heat until just soft; 2 to 3 minutes. Stir in mushrooms; cook and stir for 2 minutes longer.

Stir in rice and chicken stock. Heat to boiling, stirring frequently. Reduce heat, cover and simmer until liquid is absorbed; 45 minutes.

Total CHO = 160 g   1 serving = 40 g CHO and
Total Calories = 920   230 calories
Serves 4

Note: If used for 6 small servings, each serving is approximately 25 g CHO and 150 calories.

RICE ITALIANO*

---

1 litre/1¾ pints chicken   1 tbsp dry mustard
   stock   400 g/14 oz brown rice
2 tsp Italian herb seasoning   25 g/1 oz pine nuts or
1 tsp Worcestershire sauce   chopped almonds

Heat chicken stock, herb seasoning, Worcestershire sauce, mustard and rice to boiling in a large saucepan, stirring once or twice. Reduce heat, cover pan tightly and cook until liquid is absorbed; about 30 minutes. Fluff rice with a fork and stir in nuts. Cover and let steam for 5 to 10 minutes.

Total CHO = 275 g   1 serving = 35 g and 190
Total Calories = 1520   calories
Serves 8

POTATO AND ONION BAKE

---

900 g/2 lb potatoes, scrubbed
 and cut into 1 cm/½ in
 slices
225 g/8 oz onions, thinly
 sliced

4 tbsp margarine
salt and freshly ground
 pepper

Very lightly oil a 2.8 litre/5 pint casserole. Alternate layers of potato and onion slices, dotting each layer with margarine and seasoning with salt and pepper. Bake in a 170°C/325°F/mark 3 oven until potatoes are tender; about 40 minutes.

Total CHO = 160 g
Total Calories = 1200
Serves 8

1 serving = 20 g CHO and
 150 calories

STUFFING*

---

175 g/6 oz onion,
 chopped
150 g/5 oz celery, diced
2 medium apples, peeled and
 diced

150 g/5 oz walnuts, chopped
225 g/8 oz packet herb
 stuffing mix
100 g/4 oz margarine,
 melted

Combine onion, celery, apples, walnuts and stuffing mix in a large bowl. Pour margarine over ingredients and mix lightly. *Yield:* enough stuffing for a 10-lb turkey or 2 roasting chickens

Total CHO = 200 g
Total Calories = 2500
Enough for 10 large or 20
 small servings

1 serving = 20 or 10 g CHO
 and 250 or 125 calories

YELLOW RICE PILAF*

---

1 medium carrot, peeled and
  very finely chopped
1 small onion, finely
  chopped
75 g/3 oz celery, thinly
  sliced

2 tbsp margarine
200 g/7 oz brown rice
550 ml/1 pint water
1½ tsp salt

Cook and stir carrot, onion and celery in margarine in a
medium saucepan until tender. Stir in rice, water and salt.
Heat to boiling. Reduce heat, cover and simmer until all liquid
is absorbed; 30–40 minutes.

Total CHO = 160 g
Total Calories = 920
Serves 8 small portions

1 serving = 20 g CHO and
  115 calories

WHITE BEANS AND TOMATOES*

---

400 g/14 oz can tomatoes
440 g/15½ oz can white
  kidney beans, drained

450 g/1 lb courgettes, thinly
  sliced
salt and freshly ground
  pepper

Empty tomatoes into a saucepan and break up with a fork. Stir
in beans and courgette. Heat to boiling. Reduce heat, cover
and simmer until courgette is crisp-tender; 10 to 15 minutes.
Season with salt and pepper.

Total CHO = 80 g
Total Calories = 480
Serves 8

1 serving = 10 g CHO and
  60 calories

Pasta and
Non-meat Main Dishes

THICK TOMATO SAUCE

175 g/6 oz onion, chopped
4 tbsp vegetable oil
3 × 400 g/14 oz canned
  tomatoes, drained and
  finely chopped

1 clove garlic, crushed
1 tsp oregano
pinch freshly ground pepper

Cook and stir onion in oil until tender. Stir in remaining ingredients. Heat to boiling, stirring frequently. Reduce heat and simmer for at least 1 hour. (Sauce becomes smoother the longer it simmers.) If desired, sauce can be puréed in a blender or food processor for smoother consistency.

Total CHO = 40 g
Total Calories = 700
Serves 4

1 serving = 10 g CHO and
  175 calories

PESTO SAUCE

---

100 g/4 oz coarsely chopped
   fresh basil; or use
   plain-leaved parsley,
   coarsely chopped plus 2
   tbsp dried basil
½ tsp freshly ground black
   pepper
1–2 tsp finely chopped garlic

½ tsp salt
25 g/1 oz pine nuts or
   walnuts, chopped
200 ml/7 fl oz olive oil
50 g/2 oz freshly grated
   Parmesan cheese

Measure all ingredients except cheese into a blender or food processor. Process until smooth. Pour into a saucepan and heat. Remove from heat; stir in cheese until blended. Serve with wholemeal pasta.

Total CHO = negligible
Total Calories = 2000
Serves 8

1 serving = negligible CHO
   and 250 calories

PASTA WITH VEGETABLES

---

200 g/7 oz wholemeal pasta
1 medium onion, sliced
2 tbsp margarine
2 medium courgettes, sliced
1 medium green pepper,
   seeded and chopped

1 medium red pepper, seeded
   and chopped
100 g/4 oz broccoli florets
25 g/1 oz grated Parmesan
   cheese

Cook pasta as directed on packet; keep warm.

   Cook and stir onion in margarine until just soft; 3 minutes. Add courgettes, green pepper, red pepper and broccoli. Cook and stir until crisp-tender and heated through; about 5 minutes.

Combine warm pasta and vegetable mixture in a large bowl; sprinkle with Parmesan cheese and toss.

Total CHO = 140 g   1 serving = 35 g CHO and
Total Calories = 1000   250 calories
Serves 4

MUSHROOM AND ALMOND PASTA

150 g/5 oz wholemeal pasta   2 tbsp margarine
225 g/8 oz mushrooms,   salt and freshly ground
   thinly sliced   pepper
100 g/4 oz flaked almonds,   50 g/2 oz grated Parmesan
   toasted   cheese
                         4 tbsp chopped parsley

Cook pasta as directed on packet; keep warm.

Cook and stir mushrooms and almonds in margarine over medium-high heat until mushrooms are soft; 4 to 5 minutes. Season with salt and pepper.

Divide warm pasta into 4 servings and top each with mushroom mixture. Sprinkle each with 2 tbsp Parmesan cheese and 1 tbsp parsley.

Total CHO = 100 g   1 serving = 25 g CHO and
Total Calories = 1500   375 calories
Serves 4

SPAGHETTI PRIMAVERA

---

200 g/7 oz wholemeal
  spaghetti
450 g/1 lb fresh broccoli
  florets
225 g/8 oz cauliflower florets
4 tbsp margarine
225 g/8 oz small firm
  tomatoes, quartered
2 cloves garlic, finely
  chopped

2 tbsp vegetable oil
½ tsp salt
1 tsp basil
pinch freshly ground pepper
50 g/2 oz grated Parmesan
  cheese
3 tbsp chopped parsley
175 ml/6 fl oz chicken stock

Cook spaghetti as directed on packet, adding broccoli and cauliflower for last 5 minutes. Drain; return spaghetti and vegetables to saucepan and add 2 tbsp margarine; toss to coat ingredients.

Cook and stir tomatoes and garlic in oil and remaining margarine for 6 minutes. Stir in salt, basil and pepper. Add tomatoes to spaghetti mixture. Stir in cheese, parsley and enough chicken stock for desired consistency. Heat, stirring frequently.

Total CHO = 160 g
Total Calories = 1720
Serves 4

1 serving = 40 g CHO and
  430 calories

CHEESE SOUFFLÉ

---

50 g/2 oz margarine
25 g/1 oz wholemeal flour
2 tsp dry mustard
pinch cayenne pepper

275 ml/½ pint skimmed milk
175 g/6 oz mature Cheddar
  cheese, coarsely grated
6 eggs, separated

Melt margarine in a saucepan over low heat. Stir in flour, mustard and cayenne pepper. Cook gently until smooth and bubbly. Remove from heat and stir in milk. Heat to boiling, stirring constantly. Boil and stir for 1 minute. Stir in cheese and heat gently until melted. Remove from heat.

Beat egg yolks until thick. Blend into cheese mixture. Cool for about 15 minutes.

Heat oven to 180°C/350°F/mark 4. Lightly oil a 25 cm/10 in soufflé dish. Beat egg whites until stiff peaks form. Stir about half the egg whites into cheese mixture. (Mixture will be foamy.) Carefully fold in remaining whites. Pour mixture into soufflé dish and bake until golden and puffed; about 25 minutes. Serve at once.

Total CHO = 30 g	1 serving = 5 g CHO and
Total Calories = 1740	290 calories
Serves 6	

FRESH VEGETABLE SOUFFLÉ

25 g/1 oz plain flour
⅛ tsp freshly ground pepper
½ tsp dill weed
½ tsp dry mustard
100 g/4 oz reduced-calorie
   mayonnaise

4 tbsp skimmed milk
225 g/8 oz finely chopped
   cooked vegetables (carrot,
   green beans, green
   pepper, sweetcorn)
4 egg whites

Heat oven to 170°C/325°F/mark 3. Lightly oil a 1.7 litre/3 pint soufflé dish. Mix flour, pepper, dill weed, mustard and mayonnaise. Stir in milk and vegetables.

Beat egg whites until stiff peaks form. Fold vegetable mixture into egg whites. Pour into soufflé dish. Bake until a knife inserted in centre comes out clean; 40 minutes. Serve immediately.

Total CHO = 40 g
Total Calories = 500
Serves 4

1 serving = 10 g CHO and
125 calories

COURGETTE AND TOMATO FLAN

Pastry for 23 cm/9 in flan
   case (page 186)
450 g/1 lb courgettes,
   trimmed and sliced
2 medium onions, thinly
   sliced and separated into
   rings
2 tbsp vegetable oil
¼ tsp garlic salt
freshly ground pepper
1 medium tomato, sliced

1 egg
275 ml/½ pint skimmed
   milk
1 tbsp Italian herb seasoning
1 tsp dry mustard
¼ tsp salt
50 g/2 oz Mozzarella cheese,
   finely chopped
25 g/1 oz grated Parmesan
   cheese

Prepare pastry. Cook and stir courgettes and onion in a large frying pan in oil until onion is tender and courgette light brown; about 5 minutes. Season with garlic salt and pepper.

Heat oven to 180°C/350°F/mark 4. Place courgette mixture in pastry-lined flan tin; top with tomato slices. Beat egg, milk, Italian seasoning, mustard and salt. Stir in Mozzarella cheese; season with pepper and pour over vegetables. Sprinkle Parmesan cheese on top. Bake for 40 to 45 minutes, until filling is set and top is brown.

Total CHO = 150 g
Total Calories = 1920
Serves 6

1 serving = 25 g CHO and
320 calories

COURGETTE CASSEROLE

---

2 egg whites
75 ml/⅛ pint skimmed milk
900 g/2 lb courgettes, diced
25 g/1 oz bran
1 medium onion, chopped

¼ tsp garlic salt
pinch freshly ground pepper
225 g/8 oz Cheddar cheese,
   grated

Heat oven to 170°C/325°F/mark 3. Lightly oil an ovenproof casserole. Beat egg white and skimmed milk in a large bowl until blended. Stir in remaining ingredients. Pour into casserole and bake for 40 minutes.

Total CHO = 40 g
Total Calories = 1200
Serves 4 (large helpings)

1 serving = 10 g CHO and
   300 calories

RATATOUILLE FLAN

Pastry for 23 cm/9 in flan
   case (page 186)
1 large onion, halved and
   thinly sliced
450 g/1 lb aubergines, peeled
   and diced
150 g/5 oz courgettes, diced
1 medium green pepper,
   seeded and chopped

2 tbsp olive oil
pinch garlic salt and freshly
   ground pepper
1 large or 2 medium
   tomatoes, blanched,
   skinned and sliced
225 g/8 oz Emmental cheese,
   coarsely grated

Prepare pastry and heat oven to 180°C/350°F/mark 4.

Cook and stir onion, aubergines, courgettes and green pepper in olive oil in a large frying pan until aubergine is tender; 8 to 10 minutes. Season with garlic salt and pepper.

Turn into pastry-lined flan tin. Place tomato slices on top and sprinkle with cheese.

Bake for 30 minutes, until pastry is cooked and cheese melted.

Total CHO = 120 g   1 serving = 10 or 20 g CHO
Total Calories = 2340   and 195 or 390 calories
Serves 12 small or 6 medium
   portions

Fish

GRILLED SALMON

50 g/2 oz unsalted
   margarine, softened
1 tbsp mustard
juice of ½ lemon
pinch cayenne pepper
1 tbsp chopped parsley

4 × 100 g/4 oz salmon
   steaks
salt and freshly ground
   pepper
1 tbsp olive oil

First make the sauce. Mix margarine, mustard, lemon juice, cayenne pepper and parsley in a small bowl. Cover and refrigerate for 1 hour.

Heat the grill to high. Season fish steaks with salt and pepper and brush with oil. Grill steaks, turning once, until fish flakes easily with a fork; about 7 minutes. Serve with sauce.

Total CHO = negligible
Total Calories = 1300
Serves 4

1 serving = negligible CHO
   and 325 calories

SOLE AMANDINE*

---

50 g/2 oz margarine
675 g/1½ lb lemon sole
  fillets
25 g/1 oz flaked almonds

1 tsp grated lemon peel
2 tsp lemon juice
parsley sprigs
lemon wedges

Melt two-thirds of margarine in a large frying pan over medium heat. Cook half the fillets at a time until golden brown; about 2 minutes on each side. Remove fish to a serving platter and keep warm.

Melt remaining margarine in the pan; cook and stir almonds, lemon peel and juice for 1 minute. Pour over fish and garnish with parsley and lemon wedges.

Total CHO = negligible
Total Calories = 990
Serves 6

1 serving = negligible CHO
  and 165 calories

CELESTIAL STEAMED FISH*

---

4 × 225 g/8 oz white fish
  (small plaice, sole or dabs)
  cleaned and wiped dry
½ tsp salt
4 × 1 cm/½ in thick slices
  fresh ginger root, cut into
  slivers

3 tbsp vegetable oil
3 tbsp soy sauce
4 spring onions, very finely
  chopped

Place fish in a steamer; sprinkle with salt and ginger. Add boiling water, cover and steam for 20 minutes. (If you do not have a steamer, place a rack in a pan large enough to hold a plate with the fish on it. Pour in enough boiling water to cover the rack. Cover and steam fish for 20 minutes.)

Place fish on a serving dish. Heat vegetable oil; pour over fish. Sprinkle on soy sauce and top with chopped onion.

Total CHO = negligible   1 serving = negligible CHO
Total Calories = 1000   and 250 calories
Serves 4

CURRIED FISH FILLETS

450 g/1 lb white fish fillets,   2 tsp cornflour
  thawed if frozen   2 tsp chopped parsley
1/2 tsp salt   1 clove garlic, finely chopped
1/4 tsp white pepper   2 tsp curry powder
225 g/8 oz tomatoes,   1/2 tsp basil
  blanched, skinned, seeded   75 g/3 oz canned sweetcorn,
  and chopped   warmed, to garnish
2–3 spring onions, sliced
275 ml/1/2 pint skimmed
  milk

Heat oven to 200°C/400°F/mark 6. Arrange fish in a single layer in a baking dish. Sprinkle with salt and pepper. Spread tomato and onion evenly on fish. Blend milk and cornflour; stir in remaining ingredients and pour mixture over fish.

Cover with foil; bake until fish flakes easily with a fork; 20 to 25 minutes. Serve garnished with sweetcorn.

Total CHO = 40 g   1 serving = 10 g CHO and
Total Calories = 500   125 calories
Serves 4

FILLET OF SOLE PEDRO

---

675 g/1½ lb sole fillets
juice of 1 lemon
salt and freshly ground
pepper
1 medium tomato, blanched,
skinned and sliced

1 tbsp margarine
lemon wedges
chopped parsley

Cover a baking sheet with foil; brush lightly with oil. Arrange fish on baking sheet and season with lemon juice, salt and pepper. Arrange tomato slices on top and dot with margarine. Bake in a 170°C/325°F/mark 3 oven until fish flakes easily with fork; 10 to 15 minutes. Remove fish to a warm serving dish and garnish with lemon wedges and parsley.

Total CHO = negligible
Total Calories = 600
Serves 6

1 serving = negligible CHO
and 100 calories

HERB-BAKED FISH FILLETS

---

450 g/1 lb firm white fish
fillets
1 tsp chopped parsley
¼ tsp thyme
salt and freshly ground
pepper
175 ml/6 fl oz chicken stock

225 g/8 oz mushrooms,
sliced
2 tsp margarine
lemon wedges
1 tomato, thinly sliced

Place fish in a lightly oiled shallow baking dish. Sprinkle with parsley, thyme, salt and pepper. Pour stock over fish. Bake in a 230°C/450°F/mark 8 oven until fish flakes easily with a fork; 15 to 20 minutes. Remove fish to a warm serving dish.

Meanwhile cook and stir mushrooms in margarine until tender and all liquid is absorbed. Surround fish with mushrooms and garnish with lemon wedges and tomato slices.

Total CHO = negligible   1 serving = negligible CHO
Total Calories = 440   and 110 calories
Serves 4

TROUT WITH GRAPES

6 × 175–200 g/6–7 oz   50 g/2 oz flaked almonds
    whole rainbow trout, split   4 spring onions, thinly sliced
    open   200 g/7 oz black grapes,
½ lemon   halved and seeded
freshly ground pepper
75 g/3 oz margarine

Line grill pan with aluminium foil. Spread fish flat, skin side down, in pan. (You may have to cook them in two batches.) Squeeze juice from half lemon on fish; season with pepper. Dot fish with half the margarine.

Heat the grill to high. Grill fish, turning once, until flesh flakes easily with a fork; 5 to 7 minutes.

Cook and stir almonds and spring onions in remaining margarine until onions are soft. Stir in grapes and heat through. Serve fish covered with grape topping.

Total CHO = 30 g   1 serving = 5 g CHO and
Total Calories = 2040   340 calories
Serves 6

TROUT WITH MUSHROOMS

---

4 × 175–200 g/6–7 oz
  whole rainbow trout,
  cleaned and heads
  removed
salt and freshly ground
  pepper
1 tbsp chervil, dill weed or
  tarragon
50 g/2 oz margarine

3–4 spring onions, thinly
  sliced
225 g/8 oz mushrooms,
  thinly sliced
red pepper sauce (Tabasco),
  optional
lemon wedges

Heat grill to high. Line grill pan with foil. Arrange fish in pan; season with salt and pepper and sprinkle with chervil. Dot each fish with a little of the margarine. Grill, turning once, until flesh flakes easily with a fork; 8 to 10 minutes.

Cook and stir spring onions in the remaining margarine for 1 minute. Add mushrooms and cook, stirring until mushrooms are soft; 2 to 3 minutes. Season with salt and pepper and, if desired, a few drops of red pepper sauce. Top fish with mushroom mixture and garnish with lemon wedges.

Total CHO = negligible
Total Calories = 1200
Serves 4

1 serving = negligible CHO
  and 300 calories

CRAB NORFOLK*

---

50 g/2 oz margarine
4 cloves garlic, crushed
2 × 200 g/7 oz cans
  crabmeat, drained and
  cartilage removed

pinch freshly ground pepper
2–3 tbsp chopped parsley
lemon wedges

Melt margarine in a small frying pan. Add garlic; cook and stir over low heat for 5 minutes. Add crabmeat; cook and stir over medium heat for 5 minutes. Remove crabmeat to a warm plate. Season with pepper and garnish with parsley and lemon wedges.

Total CHO = negligible   1 serving = negligible CHO
Total Calories = 600   and 150 calories
Serves 4

ITALIAN BAKED FISH FILLETS*

675 g/1½ lb white fish fillets   50 g/2 oz grated Parmesan
75 g/3 oz wholemeal   cheese
   bread, crumbed and dried   2 tbsp chopped parsley
¼ tsp pepper   ¼ tsp garlic powder
¼ tsp salt   2 eggs
½ tsp oregano or Italian   50 g/2 oz wholemeal flour
   herb seasoning   parsley sprigs
                                     lemon wedges

Heat oven to 180°C/350°F/mark 4. If fillets are large, cut into serving pieces. Mix breadcrumbs, pepper, salt, oregano, cheese, parsley and garlic powder in a roasting tin. Beat eggs in a shallow bowl. Dip fish into flour and then into egg and coat with crumb mixture.

Place fish on a lightly oiled baking sheet. Bake until flesh flakes easily with a fork; 10 to 15 minutes. Remove to a warm serving dish and garnish with parsley sprigs and lemon wedges.

Total CHO = 60 g   1 serving = 10 g CHO and
Total Calories = 1020   170 calories
Serves 6

PIQUANT COD STEAKS

---

4 × 175 g/6 oz cod steaks (or 1 tbsp margarine
   other firm fish steaks)   pinch salt and freshly
juice of 2 lemons   ground pepper
1 tsp grated fresh ginger root chopped parsley
   or 2 tsp ground ginger lemon wedges

Arrange fish in a shallow baking dish. Mix lemon juice and ginger; pour over fish. Marinate for 30 to 40 minutes, turning fish several times.

Heat the grill to high. Lightly oil the grill pan. Arrange fish in the pan, dot each with margarine and season with salt and pepper. Grill for about 10 minutes, turning once, until flesh flakes easily with a fork. Garnish with parsley and lemon wedges.

Total CHO = negligible   1 serving = negligible CHO
Total Calories = 600   and 150 calories
Serves 4

OVEN-BAKED HADDOCK

Courgette and Leek Sauté   1 tsp oregano
   (overleaf)   1 tsp chopped parsley
900 g/2 lb haddock fillets,   ¼ tsp garlic powder
   skinned   1 tbsp sesame seeds
75 g/3 oz wholemeal   25 g/1 oz wholemeal flour
   bread, crumbed and dried 1 egg, beaten
25 g/1 oz grated Parmesan
   cheese

Prepare Courgette and Leek Sauté; keep warm.
Heat oven to 200°C/400°F/mark 6. Cut fish into 6 serving pieces. Mix breadcrumbs, cheese, oregano, parsley, garlic powder and sesame seeds in a shallow dish. Coat fish with flour, then dip into egg and cover with breadcrumb mixture. Place on a baking sheet.
Bake until flesh flakes easily with a fork; 10 to 12 minutes. Remove fish to a warm dish and surround with Courgette and Leek Sauté.

Courgette and Leek Sauté

3 tbsp olive oil
1 leek, cut into 6 mm/¼ in
   slices
450 g/1 lb courgettes, cut
   into 1 cm/½ in slices

1 medium red pepper, seeded
   and cut into 2.5 cm/1 in
   strips

Heat oil in a large pan. Cook and stir vegetables until tender; 8 to 10 minutes.

Total CHO = 60 g
Total Calories = 1680
Serves 6

1 serving = 10 g CHO and
   280 calories

Meat

ALL-DAY OVEN STEW*

---

900 g/2 lb lean stewing
   meat, cubed
225 g/8 oz celery stalks, cut
   into 4 cm/1½ in pieces
225 g/8 oz carrots, peeled
   and cut into 4 cm/1½ in
   pieces
225 g/8 oz onions, quartered

675 g/1½ lb potatoes,
   quartered
800 g/28 oz can tomatoes,
   processed or sieved
1 tbsp salt
pinch freshly ground pepper
1 tbsp cornflour

Heat oven to 130°C/250°F/mark ½. Combine meat, celery,
carrots, onions and potatoes in a large casserole. Mix tomatoes, salt, pepper and cornflour; pour into casserole. Cover
and cook for 5 hours.

Total CHO = 180 g
Total Calories = 2100
Serves 6

1 serving = 30 g CHO and
   350 calories

HIGH-FIBRE MEAT LOAF

---

450 g/1 lb lean minced beef
275 ml/½ pint tomato juice
75 g/3 oz porridge oats
2 tbsp bran
75 g/3 oz carrot, peeled and
  finely diced

1 egg white, beaten
1 small onion, chopped
½ tsp salt
pinch freshly ground pepper
¼ tsp dry mustard

Heat oven to 180°C/350°F/mark 4. Measure all ingredients into a large bowl and mix. Press mixture into a loaf tin and bake for 1 hour. Allow loaf to stand for 5 minutes before slicing.

Total CHO = 80 g
Total Calories = 1200
Serves 8

1 serving = 10 g CHO and
  150 calories

FLANK STEAK AND PEPPERS

---

450 g/1 lb very lean beef
  flank or skirt, scored
1 tsp garlic salt
pinch freshly ground
  pepper
3 tbsp vegetable oil

2 tbsp wine vinegar
½ tsp garlic powder
½ tsp dry mustard
1 tsp thyme
Pepper Topping (below)

Season steak with garlic salt and pepper. Place in a shallow bowl. Mix oil, vinegar, garlic powder, mustard and thyme. Pour over steak. Cover and refrigerate, turning occasionally, for 3 to 4 hours or overnight.

Prepare Pepper Topping and keep it warm.

Heat grill to high. Grill steak for about 5 minutes. Turn and grill for about 5 minutes more. Remove to a heated serving dish.

Cut meat across grain at a slanted angle, into thin slices. Serve covered with Pepper Topping.

Pepper Topping

1 large onion, thinly sliced
1 medium green pepper,
    seeded and thinly sliced

1 medium red pepper, seeded
    and thinly sliced
1 tbsp vegetable oil

Cook and stir vegetables in oil over medium heat until onion is tender.

Total CHO = 10 g
Total Calories = 1400
Serves 4

1 serving = negligible CHO
    and 350 calories

MOCK STEAK BÉARNAISE

450 g/1 lb lean minced beef
4 large slices wholemeal
    bread (150 g/5 oz)
1 tbsp margarine

1 medium tomato, sliced
½ quantity Béarnaise Sauce
    (below)
parsley sprigs

Shape meat into 4 patties, each about 4 cm/3 in across and 2.5 cm/1 in thick. Heat the grill to high and grill them for 3 to 4 minutes on each side for rare, 5 to 7 minutes for medium.

Remove crusts from bread and cut into four 8 cm/3 in circles. Spread with margarine; toast in a large frying pan. Place a tomato slice on each toast round; then top with a meat patty and Béarnaise Sauce. Garnish with a parsley sprig.

Total CHO = 60 g   1 serving = 15 g CHO and
Total Calories = 1560   390 calories
Serves 4

Béarnaise Sauce

3 egg yolks   ¼ tsp tarragon
2 tsp tarragon vinegar   50 g/2 oz margarine, melted
¼ tsp salt

Put egg yolks, vinegar, salt and tarragon in a blender on high
speed and process until smooth; about 2 seconds. Add the hot
margarine drop by drop, continuing to blend on high speed.

Total CHO = negligible   Total Calories = 580

ONE-POT DINNER

2 tbsp vegetable oil   1 bay leaf
450 g/1 lb lean beef, flank or   225 g/8 oz whole green
   skirt, scored   beans, cut into 2.5 cm/1 in
1 medium onion, chopped   pieces
150 ml/¼ pint beef stock   450 g/1 lb potatoes,
2 cloves garlic, crushed   quartered
1 tsp red pepper sauce   450 g/1 lb carrots, peeled
   (Tabasco)   and cut into 5 cm/2 in
½ tsp oregano   pieces
½ tsp salt

Heat oil in a large heavy saucepan; brown meat on both sides
over medium heat. Add onion; cook and stir until tender. Stir
in stock, garlic, pepper sauce, oregano, salt and bay leaf; heat

to boiling. Reduce heat, cover and simmer for 1 hour. Add water or more stock if necessary. Add beans, potatoes and carrots. Cover and cook over medium heat until potatoes are tender; about 30 minutes. Remove bay leaf before serving.

Total CHO = 100 g
Total Calories = 1600
Serves 4

1 serving = 25 g and 400 calories

STEAK DIANE

75 g/3 oz sliced mushrooms
2 tbsp finely chopped onion
1 clove garlic, crushed
⅛ tsp salt
1 tsp lemon juice

1 tsp Worcestershire sauce
5 tbsp margarine
2 tbsp chopped parsley
450 g/1 lb lean beef fillet,
    trimmed and cut into 8
    slices

Cook and stir mushrooms, onion and seasonings in 3 tbsp margarine until mushrooms are tender. Stir in parsley and keep warm.

Melt 2 tbsp margarine in a large frying pan. Cook meat in margarine, turning once, over medium-high heat until medium done; 3 to 4 minutes on each side. Serve with mushrooms.

Total CHO = negligible
Total Calories = 1200
Serves 4

1 serving = negligible CHO and 300 calories

BEEF WITH BROCCOLI

---

*450 g/1 lb lean beef flank or
  skirt, shredded (see below)*
*2 cloves garlic, finely
  chopped*
1 tsp grated fresh ginger root
2 tbsp vegetable oil

*450 g/1 lb broccoli,
  separated into small
  florets and stems, thinly
  sliced*
1½ tsp cornflour
3 tbsp water
25 ml/1 fl oz soy sauce

Combine shredded meat, garlic and ginger root in a bowl and toss. Let stand for 30 minutes.

Heat a wok or large frying pan; add oil and rotate pan to coat. Add meat and stir-fry until brown; 2 to 3 minutes. Add broccoli and stir-fry until crisp-tender; 1 to 2 minutes. Mix cornflour, water and soy sauce; stir into meat mixture. Cook, stirring constantly, until mixture boils and thickens. Then cook and stir for another minute.

To shred meat: cut it with grain into long strips, about 5 cm/2 in wide. Cut each strip across grain into 3 mm/⅛ in slices. Stack slices and cut into thin strips.

Total CHO = 20 g
Total Calories = 1200
Serves 6

1 serving = negligible CHO
  and 200 calories

BRISKET WITH APPLES AND CARAWAY

---

*350 g/12 oz cooking apples,
  unpeeled and sliced*
350 g/12 oz onions, sliced
*25 g/1 oz fresh rye
  bread, crumbed and dried*
2 tsp caraway seeds

*1.4 kg/3 lb lean beef brisket,
  trimmed of visible fat*
2 tbsp wholemeal flour
¼ tsp black pepper
1 tbsp red wine vinegar

Arrange half the apple slices, half the onion slices, the bread-crumbs and 1 tsp caraway seeds in a casserole. Place meat in casserole; sprinkle with flour and pepper. Cover meat with remaining apple and onion slices and caraway seeds. Cover tightly and bake in a 180°C/350°F/mark 4 oven until meat is tender; about 2 hours.

Remove meat to a warm platter. Skim fat from liquid. Pour apple and onion mixture into a food mill, blender or food processor and work until smooth. Stir in vinegar and, if desired, season with pepper. If necessary, thin sauce with water.

Cut meat into thin slices; arrange slices on a serving dish. Heat puréed sauce to boiling and pour over meat.

Total CHO = 60 g   1 serving = 5 g CHO and
Total Calories = 2820   235 calories
Serves 12

VEAL PICCATA

675 g/1½ lb veal escalopes   *8 thin lemon slices*
freshly ground pepper   *75 ml/⅛ pint dry white wine*
2 tbsp margarine   *or vermouth*
1½ tsp tarragon   *2 tbsp chopped parsley*

Place escalopes between sheets of greaseproof paper and pound carefully until 6 mm/¼ in thick with a rolling pin or meat hammer. Season with pepper.

Melt margarine in a large frying pan. Brown 3 or 4 escalopes at a time over medium-high heat; turn and brown other side. Remove to a warm dish. Add tarragon, lemon slices and wine to pan and heat. Pour over veal and sprinkle parsley on top.

Total CHO = negligible
Total Calories = 1020
Serves 6

1 serving = negligible CHO
and 170 calories

VEAL MARSALA WITH PROSCIUTTO

675 g/1½ lb boneless veal
   steak
2 tbsp wholemeal flour
3 tbsp olive oil
50 g/2 oz margarine
1 small onion, finely
   chopped
1 clove garlic, crushed
225 g/8 oz mushrooms,
   thinly sliced
1 tsp lemon juice

175 ml/6 fl oz Marsala wine
3 tbsp chopped parsley
1 tbsp basil
100 g/4 oz prosciutto (raw
   Italian ham), thinly sliced
   and cut into 1 cm/½ in
   strips
salt and pinch freshly
   ground pepper

Cut veal into 6 serving pieces. Coat with flour; pound with a meat hammer or rolling pin until 6 mm/¼ in thick. Heat oil and margarine in a large frying pan. Cook veal until tender and brown; about 4 minutes on each side. Remove to a warm dish and keep warm.

Cook and stir onion and garlic in the pan until onion is tender; 3 to 4 minutes. Add mushrooms and lemon juice; cook and stir over medium heat until mushrooms are soft. Stir in wine, parsley, basil and prosciutto. Heat to boiling. Reduce heat and simmer for 1 minute. Season with salt and pepper. Place meat in sauce and heat through for 2 to 3 minutes.

Total CHO = 20 g
Total Calories = 1800
Serves 6

1 serving = negligible CHO
and 300 calories

VEAL WITH MUSHROOMS

---

4 small boneless veal steaks
  or cutlets (total weight
  450 g/1 lb)
salt and freshly ground
  pepper
2 tbsp wholemeal flour
2 tbsp olive oil

150 ml/¼ pint extra dry
  white vermouth or Italian
  dry white wine
100 g/4 oz mushrooms,
  thinly sliced
chopped parsley
lemon wedges

Pound meat with a meat hammer or rolling pin until 6 mm/¼ in thick. Season with salt and pepper and coat with flour.

Heat oil in a large frying pan and brown meat over medium-high heat; 3 to 4 minutes on each side. Pour wine into pan; heat to boiling. Reduce heat, cover and simmer for 2 to 3 minutes. Spread mushrooms over meat in pan, cover and simmer for 2 to 3 minutes more.

Remove meat and mushrooms to a warm serving dish and pour sauce over. Garnish with parsley and lemon wedges.

Total CHO = 10 g
Total Calories = 900
Serves 4

1 serving = negligible CHO
  and 225 calories

HAM AND CHEESE QUICHE*

---

unbaked 23 cm/9 in pastry
  case, chilled
150 g/5 oz ham, diced
225 g/8 oz Emmental cheese,
  grated

3 eggs, beaten
150 ml/¼ pint chicken stock
142 ml/5 fl oz single cream

Heat oven to 230°C/450°F/mark 8. Prick bottom and side of pastry case with a fork. Bake for 5 minutes. Remove from oven.

Layer ham and cheese in pastry case. Mix eggs, chicken stock and cream; pour into pastry case. Bake for 10 minutes. Reduce oven temperature to 180°C/350°F/mark 4 and bake until a knife inserted in centre of quiche comes out clean; 20 to 25 minutes.

Total CHO = 90 g
Total Calories = 2550
Serves 6

1 serving = 15 g CHO and 425 calories

CHINESE-STYLE PORK*

2 tbsp vegetable oil
175 g/6 oz lean pork slices
  (about 6 mm/¼ in thick
  and 8 cm/3 in long)
275 ml/½ pint chicken stock
450 g/1 lb mange-tout peas

200 g/7 oz sliced water
  chestnuts
1 tbsp cornflour
1 tbsp water
2 tbsp soy sauce

Heat a wok or large frying pan until 1 or 2 drops water skitter around when sprinkled in. Add oil; rotate to coat side of pan. Add pork and stir-fry until it is no longer pink. Add stock, cover and cook over medium heat for 3 minutes. Add peas and water chestnuts; stir-fry for 1 minute. Mix cornflour, water and soy sauce; stir into meat mixture. Cook and stir over medium heat until mixture thickens and boils. Serve at once.

Total CHO = 60 g
Total Calories = 840
Serves 6

1 serving = 10 g CHO and 140 calories

PORK STEAKS DIJON*

---

6 × 100 g/4 oz boned pork
    steaks
50 g/2 oz wholemeal flour
1 egg

4 tbsp Dijon mustard
3 tbsp skimmed milk
75 g/3 oz fresh wholemeal
    bread, crumbed and dried

Lightly oil a baking tin. Coat pork lightly with flour. Beat egg, milk and mustard in a shallow bowl until blended. Dip pork in mustard mixture and lightly coat with breadcrumbs. Arrange in baking tin. Bake in a 180°C/350°F/mark 4 oven until brown and tender; 1 hour.

Total CHO = 60 g
Total Calories = 1500
Serves 6

1 serving = 10 g CHO and
    250 calories

PORK CUTLETS

---

50 g/2 oz wholemeal flour
1 tsp dry mustard
1 tsp paprika
6 × 100 g/4 oz boneless pork
    steaks or cutlets
3 tbsp vegetable oil
1 egg
2 tbsp skimmed milk
75 g/3 oz fresh wholemeal
    bread, crumbed and dried

1 tbsp margarine
2 tbsp wholemeal flour
1 tsp dill weed
175 ml/6 fl oz chicken stock
150 g/5.3 oz pot low-fat
    natural yogurt
2 tbsp spicy mustard

Mix the flour, dry mustard and paprika. Coat meat with flour mixture; pound with a meat hammer or rolling pin until 6 mm/¼ in thick. Heat oil in a large frying pan. Beat egg and milk until blended. Dip meat into egg, then coat with crumbs. Cook meat in oil until brown and tender; 2 to 3 minutes on each side. (Do not crowd meat in pan; cook in batches if necessary.) Remove meat to a warm dish and keep warm.

Melt the margarine in the pan. Blend in 2 tbsp flour and dill weed. Cook over low heat, stirring constantly, until smooth. Stir in stock. Heat to boiling, stirring constantly. Reduce heat to low; stir in yogurt and mustard, and heat. (Do not allow to boil.) Pour into a sauceboat.

Total CHO = 90 g   1 serving = 15 g CHO and
Total Calories = 2160   360 calories
Serves 6

BEEF OR LAMB SHISH KEBABS

Meat-basting Sauce   *6 small tomatoes, halved*
  (below)   *6 mushroom caps*
175 g/6 oz lean beef or lamb, *1 medium green pepper,*
  cubed   *seeded and cut into 2.5*
2 small onions, quartered   *cm/1 in pieces*

Prepare Meat-basting Sauce. Place meat in a deep bowl; pour sauce over and refrigerate for at least 3 hours, turning meat occasionally. (Can be refrigerated for up to 24 hours.)

Drain meat well, reserving sauce. Alternate meat, onion quarters, tomato halves, mushrooms and green pepper pieces on flat skewers.

Heat grill to high and grill kebabs, turning and lightly basting occasionally with reserved sauce, until cooked to taste.

Total CHO = 10 g

1 serving = negligible CHO

Total Calories = 660

and 220 calories

Serves 3

Note: Less than one-fifth of the Meat-basting Sauce will adhere to the meat.

Meat-basting Sauce

275 ml/½ pint dry red wine
200 ml/7 fl oz vegetable oil
4 tbsp wine vinegar

2 medium onions, chopped
2 cloves garlic, split
⅛ tsp rosemary
⅛ tsp cayenne pepper

Shake all ingredients in a screw-top jar.

Total CHO = 10 g

Total Calories = 2000

Poultry

CHICKEN AND ALMONDS*

450 g/1 lb skinned, boned and diced chicken	4 tbsp vegetable oil
½ tsp salt	50 g/2 oz flaked almonds
¼ tsp freshly ground pepper	75 g/3 oz mushrooms, thinly sliced
2 tsp cornflour	150 ml/¼ pint chicken stock
2 tsp soy sauce	3 spring onions, thinly sliced
1 egg white	

Place chicken in a medium bowl. Add salt, pepper, cornflour, soy sauce, egg white and 1 tbsp of oil; mix thoroughly. Let stand for 30 minutes.

Heat a wok or large frying pan. Add remaining oil and rotate pan to coat. Add almonds; stir-fry until golden. Remove with a slotted spoon on to a paper towel. Add one-third of the chicken; stir-fry until tender (do not overcook). Remove from pan and drain on a paper towel. Stir-fry remaining chicken, half at a time, until tender. Remove from pan and drain on paper towel.

Drain all but 1 tbsp oil from pan; add mushrooms and stir-fry for 30 seconds. Add chicken stock and chicken; heat to boiling, stirring constantly. Remove to a serving dish and sprinkle almonds and spring onions on top.

Total CHO = 15 g
Total Calories = 1440
Serves 6

1 serving = negligible CHO
and 240 calories

BAKED LEMON CHICKEN

900 g/2 lb chicken pieces
1 clove garlic, crushed
juice of 1 large lemon

3 tbsp vegetable oil
chopped parsley
tomato slices

Place chicken in a glass or ceramic bowl. Sprinkle with garlic and pour on lemon juice and oil. Turn chicken to coat both sides. Cover and refrigerate for several hours or overnight, turning occasionally.

Heat oven to 180°C/350°F/mark 4. Remove chicken from marinade; place on a rack in a roasting tin, skin side up. Bake until tender and golden-brown; 35 to 40 minutes. (Alternatively, grill on medium heat.) Remove to a warm dish and garnish with parsley and tomatoes.

Total CHO = negligible
Total Calories = 1000
Serves 4

1 serving = negligible CHO
and 250 calories

CHICKEN WITH TOMATO*

---

175 g/6 oz boned white
  chicken
1 tbsp cornflour
2 tbsp soy sauce
1 tbsp dry sherry
2 tbsp vegetable oil
1 medium onion, thinly
  sliced

4 tbsp chicken stock
¼ tsp salt
2 medium tomatoes,
  blanched, skinned and cut
  into wedges

Cut chicken into 1 cm/½ in strips. Mix cornflour, soy sauce and sherry in a medium bowl. Add chicken and toss to coat all pieces. Marinate chicken in mixture for 20 minutes, tossing occasionally.

Heat oil in a wok or frying pan. Add chicken; stir-fry for 3 to 4 minutes. Add onion slices, and stir-fry for 3 minutes more. Stir in chicken stock and salt and heat to boiling. Mix tomato wedges in carefully and heat.

Total CHO = 20 g
Total Calories = 580
Serves 4

1 serving = 5 g CHO and
  145 calories

SAUTÉED CHICKEN DIJONNAISE

---

2 tbsp margarine
1 tbsp vegetable oil
4 × 100 g/4 oz boned
  chicken breast halves,
  pounded flat
75 g/3 oz wholemeal flour
150 ml/¼ pint dry vermouth

2 tbsp mustard
75 ml/⅛ pint single cream
salt and freshly ground
  pepper
2 tbsp drained capers

Heat margarine and oil in a large frying pan until very hot. Coat both sides of chicken portions with flour. Cook one at a time in the hot fat until brown on both sides. Remove to a warm plate and keep warm.

Pour wine into pan; cook over low heat for 2 minutes, scraping up loose brown bits. Stir in mustard and cream; cook for 2 minutes. Season with salt and pepper. Add chicken to sauce, turning once to coat. Turn onto a serving dish and sprinkle with capers.

Total CHO = 60 g   1 serving = 15 g CHO and
Total Calories = 1400   350 calories
Serves 4

CHICKEN WITH WALNUTS*

3 tbsp cornflour
2 tbsp dry sherry
225 g/8 oz boned white chicken cut into 2.5 cm/1 in cubes
3 tbsp vegetable oil
100 g/4 oz blanched walnut halves

1 tbsp chopped fresh ginger root
100 g/4 oz drained bamboo shoots, diced
1 small can mushrooms, drained (reserve liquid)
4 tbsp chicken stock

Combine cornflour and sherry in a medium bowl. Add chicken and toss to coat cubes. Cover and refrigerate for 20 minutes.

Heat wok or large frying pan until 1 or 2 drops of water sprinkled in pan skitter around. Add 1 tbsp oil; rotate pan to coat sides. Add walnuts; stir-fry until brown. Remove walnuts and set aside. Add ginger to pan; stir-fry for 1 minute. Add remaining oil and chicken; stir-fry until chicken turns white. Stir in bamboo shoots, mushrooms, 3 tbsp reserved mushroom liquid and chicken stock. Cover and cook over medium heat for about 3 minutes. Stir in walnuts and serve at once.

Total CHO = 40 g   1 serving = 10 g CHO and
Total Calories = 1440   360 calories
Serves 4

ONION-SMOTHERED CHICKEN*

1.4 kg/3 lb roasting chicken,   75 ml/⅛ pint soy sauce
   cut into 6 pieces   275 ml/½ pint boiling water
4 tbsp skimmed milk   5 cm/2 in piece fresh ginger
25 g/1 oz wholemeal flour   root, diced
3 tbsp vegetable oil
3 medium onions, sliced

Heat oven to 180°C/350°F/mark 4. Dip chicken into milk, then coat with flour. Heat 2 tbsp oil in a large frying pan. Cook chicken in oil over medium heat until brown on both sides. Arrange in a roasting tin.

Add remaining tbsp oil to pan; cook and stir onion until tender. Stir in soy sauce, water and ginger and heat to boiling. Pour over chicken. Cover tightly and bake until very tender; about 45 minutes. Serve with brown rice.

Total CHO = 30 g   1 serving = 5 g CHO and
Total Calories = 1350   225 calories
Serves 6

LEMON CHICKEN

1.1 kg/2½ lb roasting
   chicken, skinned and
   jointed
4 tbsp lemon juice
1 tbsp vegetable oil
½ tsp dry mustard

¼ tsp rosemary
¼ tsp thyme
¼ tsp marjoram
¼ tsp sesame seeds
¼ tsp pepper

Heat oven to 150°C/300°F/mark 2. Arrange chicken in a lightly oiled roasting tin. Mix remaining ingredients; brush part of mixture on chicken. Bake uncovered for 1 hour, brushing frequently with remaining mixture. Increase oven temperature to maximum and bake for 15 minutes more.

Total CHO = negligible
Total Calories = 1500
Serves 4

1 serving = negligible CHO
   and 375 calories

CHICKEN MARSALA*

2 tbsp margarine
3 × 225 g/8 oz boned and
   skinned chicken breasts,
   cut into halves

300 g/10½ oz can cream of
   chicken soup
75 ml/⅛ pint Marsala wine
3 tbsp chopped parsley

Melt margarine in a large frying pan. Cook chicken over medium-high heat, turning to brown both sides; about 15 minutes. Remove chicken to a baking dish. Blend soup and wine; pour over chicken. Bake in a 170°C/325°F/mark 3 oven until chicken is tender; about 30 minutes. Garnish with parsley.

Total CHO = 30 g   1 serving = 5 g CHO and
Total Calories = 1260   210 calories
Serves 6

CHICKEN WITH PEPPERS

---

900 g/2 lb boned chicken   *1 small green pepper, seeded*
50 g/2 oz wholemeal flour   *and cut into 2.5 cm/1 in*
2 tbsp margarine   *narrow strips*
1 tbsp vegetable oil   *1 small red pepper, seeded*
150 ml/¼ pint dry white   *and cut into 2.5 cm/1 in*
  wine   *narrow strips*
1 tsp lemon juice   *1 lemon, thinly sliced*

Remove skin from chicken. Coat with flour and place between 2 pieces of cling film. Pound with a meat hammer or rolling pin until 6 mm/¼ in thick, being careful not to tear meat.

Heat margarine and oil in a large frying pan until margarine is melted. Cook a few pieces of chicken at a time until golden brown, turning once. Drain and keep warm.

Return browned chicken to pan; pour wine and lemon juice over. Heat to boiling. Reduce heat, cover and simmer until chicken is tender; about 5 minutes. Add peppers and lemon slices, cover and simmer for 5 minutes more.

Total CHO = 40 g   1 serving = 5 g CHO and
Total Calories = 1760   220 calories
Serves 8

MILANESE CHICKEN*

75 g/3 oz fresh wholemeal
   bread, crumbed, dried and
   seasoned
2 tbsp grated Parmesan
   cheese
4 × 100 g/4 oz boned and
   skinned chicken breast
   halves
2–3 spring onions, chopped
2 tbsp margarine

25 g/1 oz wholemeal flour
275 ml/½ pint skimmed
   milk
2 tbsp bran
275 g/10 oz frozen chopped
   spinach, thawed and
   drained
50 g/2 oz thinly sliced lean
   boiled ham, diced

Heat oven to 170°C/325°F/mark 3. Lightly oil a shallow baking dish. Mix breadcrumbs and cheese; coat chicken with mixture, reserving 2 tbsp for topping. Arrange chicken in baking dish.

Cook and stir spring onions in margarine until tender. Stir in flour; cook over low heat until bubbly. Stir in milk. Heat to boiling, stirring constantly. Boil and stir, for 1 minute. Stir in bran, spinach and ham. Pour ham mixture over chicken. Sprinkle reserved crumb mixture on top. Bake until bubbly; 30 to 40 minutes.

Total CHO = 80 g
Total Calories = 1280
Serves 4

1 serving = 20 g CHO and
   320 calories

MEDITERRANEAN CHICKEN*

1 tbsp margarine
1 tbsp vegetable oil
675 g/1½ lb boneless
   chicken breast, cut into 1
   cm/½ in cubes
50 g/2 oz can anchovies,
   drained and chopped
1 small onion, chopped
100 g/4 oz mushrooms,
   sliced

1 small green pepper, seeded
   and chopped
½ tsp salt
¼ tsp cayenne pepper
   (optional)
50 g/2 oz pitted black olives
75 ml/⅛ pint dry white wine
800 g/28 oz can tomatoes,
   sieved

Heat margarine and oil in a large frying pan. Add chicken; cook and stir until light brown. Remove chicken from pan. Add anchovies, onion, mushroom, green pepper, salt, cayenne pepper and olives; cook, stirring occasionally, for 5 minutes. Stir in wine, tomatoes and chicken. Heat to boiling. Reduce heat and simmer for 30 minutes.

Serve chicken mixture on hot spaghetti or with creamed potatoes or boiled brown rice.

Total CHO = 30 g
Total Calories = 1410
Serves 6

1 serving = 5 g CHO and
   235 calories

LEBANESE CHICKEN AND RICE

3 × 225 g/8 oz boned and skinned chicken breasts
1 bay leaf
½ tsp coriander
225 g/8 oz lean minced lamb
50 g/2 oz chopped almonds, lightly toasted

200 g/7 oz brown rice
1 tsp salt
pinch freshly ground pepper
¼ tsp allspice
2 tbsp margarine
3 tbsp chopped parsley

Place chicken in a large frying pan. Add bay leaf and coriander and just enough water to cover chicken. Heat to boiling then reduce heat and simmer until chicken is very tender; 10 to 15 minutes. Remove from heat and cool chicken in stock.

Cut cooled chicken into 5 cm/2 in pieces; reserve stock.

Cook and stir lamb in a non-stick saucepan until light brown. Stir in almonds, rice, salt, pepper, allspice, margarine and 450 ml/¾ pint reserved stock. Heat to boiling. Reduce heat, cover and simmer until all liquid is absorbed; about 20 minutes. Stir in chicken and heat through. Season with salt and pepper and garnish with parsley.

Total CHO = 150 g
Total Calories = 2400
Serves 6

1 serving = 25 g CHO and 400 calories

CHICKEN WITH CURRIED RICE AND ALMONDS

200 g/7 oz brown rice
1 tbsp curry powder
2 tsp dry mustard
2 tbsp snipped chives

100 g/4 oz flaked almonds
425 ml/¾ pint chicken stock
1.6 kg/3½ lb chicken pieces, skinned (8 pieces)

Heat oven to 170°C/325°F/mark 3. Mix rice, curry powder, mustard, chives and almonds in an ungreased baking dish. Heat chicken stock to boiling. Stir into rice mixture. Arrange chicken pieces on top and cover tightly. Bake until chicken is tender and liquid is absorbed; about 1 hour.

Total CHO = 160 g   1 serving = 20 g CHO and
Total Calories = 2160   270 calories
Serves 8

Desserts

GRAPES AND PINEAPPLE IN SOUR CREAM

350 g/12 oz seedless green grapes, washed
225 g/8 oz can pineapple chunks in natural juice, drained

75 ml/⅛ pint sour cream

Combine grapes and pineapple chunks. Pour sour cream over fruits and toss. Refrigerate until ready to serve.

Total CHO = 80 g
Total Calories = 480
Serves 4

1 serving = 20 g CHO and
120 calories

ORANGE SNOW

2 tsp/1 envelope gelatine
150 ml/¼ pint water
200 ml/7 fl oz unsweetened orange juice
450 g/1 lb fresh orange segments, chopped

1 tbsp lemon juice
non-nutritive intense sweetener (optional)
2 egg whites
orange slices and whole strawberries

Put gelatine in a small saucepan. Stir in water and heat to boiling. Remove from heat; stir in orange juice, orange segments, lemon juice and intense sweetener to taste. Refrigerate until thickened.

Beat egg whites until stiff peaks form. Beat gelatine/orange mixture until frothy. Fold gelatine mixture into egg whites. Pour into a 1 litre/2 pint mould. Refrigerate until set. Unmould and, if desired, garnish with orange slices and whole strawberries.

Total CHO = 60 g
Total Calories = 300
Serves 6

1 serving = 10 g CHO and
50 calories

FRESH MELON SORBET

2 tsp/1 envelope gelatine
25 g/1 oz sugar
150 ml/¼ pint water
4 tbsp lemon juice
225 ml/8 fl oz water

675 g/1½ lb ripe honeydew
melon flesh, cubed; or 1.1
kg/2½ lb whole honeydew
melon, peeled, seeded and
chopped

Mix gelatine and sugar in a small saucepan. Stir in 150 ml/¼ pint water and heat to boiling, stirring until sugar is dissolved. Remove from heat. Stir in lemon juice and cool.

Pour 250 ml/8 fl oz water into a blender. Add melon cubes and blend until smooth. Stir into gelatine mixture. Pour into a small loaf tin and freeze until almost firm.

Remove from freezer; place in a bowl and beat until mushy and thick. Return to loaf tin and freeze until firm.

Total CHO = 60 g
Total Calories = 300
Serves 12

1 serving = 5 g CHO and 25
calories

SPICY APPLE TARTS

---

8 baked pastry cases (below)
25 g/1 oz hazelnuts, finely
  chopped
1.1 kg/2½ lb cooking apples,
  washed, cored and diced
  (do not peel)

1 tsp grated lemon peel
juice of 1 lemon
3 tbsp honey
1½ tsp ground cinnamon
¼ tsp ground cloves
non-nutritive intense
  sweetener to taste
  (optional)

For pastry cases, prepare standard pie pastry for 20 or 23 cm/8 or 9 in one-crust pie (page 186) except that, before mixing in water, add the hazelnuts. Roll pastry out to about 6 mm/¼ in thick. Cut into 8 rounds, about 14 cm/5½ in across, to fit into large patty tins. Prick pastry with a fork. Bake in a 230°C/450°F/mark 8 oven for 8 to 10 minutes. Cool.

Combine remaining ingredients, except sweetener, in a large saucepan. Cook over medium heat, stirring occasionally, until apples have softened but still retain their shape. Cool slightly. Taste and add sweetener if required. Spoon into pastry cases and serve.

Total CHO = 240 g
Total Calories = 1600
Makes 8

1 tart = 30 g CHO and 200
  calories

STRAWBERRY RICE

---

450 g/1 lb strawberries
425 ml/¾ pint skimmed
    milk
50 g/2 oz short-grain rice
1 tbsp lemon juice
2 tbsp water
2 tsp/1 envelope gelatine
2 egg yolks, beaten

non-nutritive intense
    sweetener to taste
    (optional)
1 egg white
2 tsp sugar
½ tsp vanilla essence
142 ml/5 fl oz pot whipping
    cream, whipped

Wash the strawberries, reserve 5 to decorate and slice the rest.

Heat milk and rice just to boiling, stirring frequently. Reduce heat to simmer; cover and cook until rice is tender; about 14 minutes.

Measure lemon juice and water into a small saucepan. Sprinkle gelatine on mixture to soften. Stir over low heat until gelatine is dissolved. Stir into hot rice and mix in egg yolks. Refrigerate, stirring occasionally. Add sweetener to taste.

Beat egg white until foamy. Beat in sugar, a little at a time; continue beating until stiff and glossy. Stir in vanilla essence. Fold into rice mixture. Fold in whipped cream and sliced strawberries. Refrigerate.

To serve, spoon into dessert dishes and top each with a reserved whole strawberry.

Total CHO = 100 g
Total Calories = 1200
Serves 5

1 serving = 20 g CHO and
    240 calories

APPLE SNOW

---

450 g/1 lb cooking apples
non-nutritive intense
   sweetener to taste

2 egg whites

Peel, core and slice apples into a saucepan. Add a small amount of water and sweetener; cover and cook over low heat until apples are soft. Turn mixture into a blender and process at high speed until smooth. Cool.

Beat egg whites until stiff. Fold into apple mixture and refrigerate.

Total CHO = 40 g
Total Calories = 160
Serves 4

1 serving = 10 g CHO and
   40 calories

BAKED APPLE RICE PUDDING

---

1 egg
225 g/8 oz cooking apples,
   peeled, cored and finely
   chopped
75 g/3 oz short-grain rice,
   cooked
75 g/3 oz stoned dates,
   chopped

ground cinnamon
2 tbsp margarine, softened
1 tsp vanilla essence
2 egg whites
apple slices dipped in lemon
   juice (optional)

Heat oven to 170°C/325°F/mark 3. Mix egg, apple, rice, dates, ½ tsp cinnamon, margarine and vanilla in a casserole or soufflé dish. Beat egg whites until stiff peaks form; fold into rice mixture. Sprinkle cinnamon on top.

Place dish in a pan of very hot water, 2.5 cm/1 in deep. Bake for about 70 minutes. Serve warm or chilled. If desired, garnish with fresh apple slices dipped in lemon juice.

Total CHO = 120 g   1 serving = 20 g CHO and
Total Calories = 840   140 calories
Serves 6

FRESH FRUIT WITH ZABAGLIONE SAUCE

2 eggs   350 g/12 oz mixed fresh fruit
150 ml/¼ pint Marsala   (e.g. whole raspberries,
   wine   sliced strawberries, peeled
non-nutritive intense   and sliced peaches and
   sweetener to taste   nectarines)

Beat eggs in the top of a double boiler until light and fluffy. Continue beating and slowly add wine. Place top of double boiler over simmering water. Cook, beating constantly, until thick and fluffy; about 20 minutes. Mixture will form soft peaks. Sweeten to taste if necessary.

Divide the fruit between 4 dessert dishes or tall wine glasses and top each with sauce.

Total CHO = 40 g   1 serving = 10 g CHO and
Total Calories = 440   110 calories
Serves 4

JAMAICAN JUMBLE

---

50 g/2 oz sliced banana
440 g/15½ oz can pineapple
  pieces in natural juice,
  finely chopped or
  processed

350 g/12 oz strawberries,
  sliced
2 tbsp Jamaican dark rum

Slice banana into a serving bowl. Stir in pineapple with juice, strawberries and rum. Cover and refrigerate.

Total CHO = 90 g
Total Calories = 420
Serves 6

1 serving = 15 g CHO and
  70 calories

EGGNOG FLUFF

---

2 eggs, separated
425 ml/¾ pint skimmed
  milk
2 tbsp honey
½ tsp nutmeg

2 tsp/1 envelope gelatine
1 tsp vanilla essence
150 g/5 oz raspberries
  (optional)

Blend egg yolks and milk in a small saucepan. Stir in honey, nutmeg and gelatine. Cook over medium-low heat, stirring constantly until mixture just boils. Remove from heat; stir in vanilla essence. Refrigerate until thickened but not set.

Beat egg whites until stiff peaks form. Beat gelatine mixture until smooth and fluffy. Fold into egg whites. Divide mixture between 6 dessert dishes and top with raspberries.

Total CHO = 60 g
Total Calories = 480
Serves 6

1 serving = 10 g CHO and
  80 calories

Miscellaneous

SHORTCRUST PASTRY

(To line a 20–23 cm/8–9 in flan case)

75 g/3 oz plain flour
50 g/2 oz wholemeal flour

75 g/3 oz unsalted
  margarine
2–4 tbsp cold water

Sieve flours into a mixing bowl. Turn residual bran back into the bowl. Cut in margarine thoroughly. Sprinkle in water, a tbsp at a time, mixing until all flour is moistened and dough comes cleanly away from side of bowl. (Use 1–2 tsp more water if necessary.) Gather dough into a ball and shape into a flattened round on a lightly floured surface. Roll out, fill and bake as directed in recipe or, to bake blind, prick bottom and sides thoroughly with a fork. Bake at 240°C/475°F/mark 9 for 8–10 minutes.

Total CHO = 100 g   Total Calories = 1000

BRAN SCONES

---

350 ml/12 fl oz buttermilk
175 g/6 oz dry bran bud
  cereal
225 g/8 oz wholemeal flour

1 tsp bicarbonate of soda
2 tsp baking powder
1/8 tsp salt
100 g/4 oz margarine

Heat oven to 180°C/350°F/mark 4. Pour buttermilk over cereal in bowl. Measure flour, bicarbonate of soda, baking powder and salt into a mixing bowl. Cut in margarine with a pastry blender or fork. Stir in buttermilk mixture.

Turn dough on to a lightly floured surface and roll to 1 cm/½ in thickness. Cut with a floured 5 cm/2 in round cutter. Bake on an oiled baking sheet until golden brown; 30 to 35 minutes.

Total CHO = 240 g
Total Calories = 2040
Makes 24 scones

1 scone = 10 g CHO and 85
  calories

HONEY WHEAT BREAD

2½ tsp dried yeast
150 ml/¼ pint warm water
  (about 43°C/110°F)
75 g/3 oz honey
1 tbsp salt
50 g/2 oz solid vegetable fat

425 ml/¾ pint warm water
350 g/12 oz stone-ground
  wholemeal flour
350 g/12 oz plain flour

Disperse yeast in 150 ml/¼ pint warm water in a large mixing bowl. Stir in honey, salt, fat, 425 ml/¾ pint warm water and the wholemeal flour. Beat until smooth. Stir in enough plain flour to make dough easy to handle.

Turn dough on to a lightly floured surface. Knead until smooth and elastic; about 10 minutes. Place in an oiled bowl; turn oiled side up. Cover; let rise in a warm place until doubled; about 1 hour. Dough is ready when, if touched, an indentation remains.

Punch down dough; divide in half. Shape each half into a loaf. Place loaves seam side down in 2 lightly oiled 450 g/1 lb loaf tins. Let rise until doubled; about 1 hour.

Heat oven to 190°C/375°F/mark 5. Bake loaves until they are golden brown and sound hollow when tapped; 40 to 45 minutes. Remove from tins; cool on a wire rack.

Total CHO = 480 g
Total Calories = 3200
Makes 2 loaves (32 slices)

1 slice = 15 g CHO and 100 calories

BEER RYE BREAD

2½ tsp dried yeast
75 ml/⅛ pint warm water
    (about 43°C/110°F)
440 ml can beer (bitter)
50 g/2 oz margarine
75 g/3 oz molasses
50 g/2 oz wheat germ

1 tbsp grated orange peel
2 tsp salt
225 g/8 oz whole rye flour
450 g/1 lb plain flour
1 egg
1 tbsp water

Disperse yeast in warm water. Heat beer, margarine and molasses until lukewarm. Pour into a mixing bowl; blend in wheat germ, orange peel, salt and yeast mixture. Mix in rye flour and enough plain flour to make dough easy to handle.

Turn dough on to a lightly floured surface. Knead until smooth and elastic; about 10 minutes. Place in an oiled bowl; turn oiled side up. Cover and let rise in a warm place until doubled; 1½ to 2 hours.

Punch down dough and knead lightly; cover and let rest for 10 minutes.

Lightly oil a baking sheet and sprinkle with flour. Shape dough into 2 rounds and place on baking sheet. Cover and let rise until doubled; about 1 hour.

Heat oven to 180°C/350°F/mark 4. Mix egg and 1 tbsp water; brush mixture on loaves. Bake loaves for 25 minutes.

Remove loaves from oven and brush again with egg glaze. Bake until loaves sound hollow when tapped; 15 to 20 minutes longer. Remove from baking sheet and cool on a wire rack.

Total CHO = 600 g   1 slice = 25 g CHO and 135
Total Calories = 3240   calories
Makes 2 loaves (24 slices)

BEER BREAD*

---

350 g/12 oz self-raising flour   *440 ml can beer, at room*
2 tbsp sugar   *temperature*
     1 tbsp margarine, melted

Heat oven to 190°C/375°F/mark 5. Lightly oil a 450 g/1 lb loaf tin. Measure flour and sugar into a mixing bowl; add enough of the beer to make a soft dough. Mix until dough comes cleanly away from side of bowl. Turn dough into a tin and bake for 40 to 45 minutes.

Remove loaf and brush top with melted margarine.

Total CHO = 300 g   1 slice = 25 g CHO and 110
Total Calories = 1320   calories
Makes 12 slices

COURGETTE MUFFINS

---

75 g/3 oz wholemeal flour
100 g/4 oz plain flour
2 tbsp bran
3 tsp baking powder
½ tsp salt
25 g/1 oz brown sugar
225 g/8 oz courgettes, grated

2 tsp grated lemon peel
1 egg
275 ml/½ pint skimmed
  milk
75 ml/⅛ pint vegetable oil

Heat oven to 200°C/400°F/mark 6. Lightly oil bottoms of 12 medium muffin tins.

Stir together in a large mixer bowl the flours, bran, baking powder and salt. Add remaining ingredients; mix at low speed, scraping bowl frequently, *just* until all the flour is moistened. Do not beat. Fill muffin tins three-quarters full.

Bake for 25 minutes. Remove from tins immediately.

Note: Recipe can be further sweetened by adding a little non-nutritive intense sweetener to the batter.

Total CHO = 180 g
Total Calories = 1620
Makes 12 muffins

1 muffin = 15 g CHO and
  135 calories

PIQUANT TOMATO SAUCE*

2–3 cloves garlic, finely
  chopped
2 tbsp olive oil
400 g/14 oz can tomatoes,
  drained (reserve juice)
1 tsp dried basil or 1 tbsp
  chopped fresh basil

1 tbsp chopped parsley
salt and freshly ground
  pepper
2 tbsp capers, drained

Cook and stir garlic in oil in a saucepan for 2 minutes. Cut tomatoes into quarters; add to garlic. Stir in reserved tomato juice, basil and parsley. Season with salt and pepper. Heat to boiling. Reduce heat and simmer for 15 minutes. Stir in capers.

Note: Serve sauce warm on grilled steak, chicken, hamburgers or veal chops. If you wish, top with chopped parsley.

Total CHO = 10 g Total Calories = 350

HOLLANDAISE SAUCE

---

2 egg yolks 100 g/4 oz margarine,
3 tbsp lemon juice melted

Put egg yolks and lemon juice into a blender. Cover and mix at high speed until smooth. Pour margarine in slowly while mixing at low speed. Mix until smooth and creamy.

Total CHO = negligible 1 serving = negligible CHO
Total Calories = 900 and 225 calories
Serves 4

MOCK HOLLANDAISE SAUCE

---

175 ml/6 fl oz reduced- pinch white pepper
  calorie mayonnaise 1 tbsp grated lemon peel
75 ml/⅛ pint skimmed milk 1 tbsp lemon juice
¼ tsp salt

Blend mayonnaise, milk, salt and pepper in a small saucepan. Cook over low heat, stirring constantly, until heated; about 3 minutes. Stir in lemon peel and juice.

Total CHO = negligible   Total Calories = 650

MEXICAN RELISH

---

450 g/1 lb firm tomatoes, diced
175 g/6 oz onion, finely chopped
150 g/5 oz red or green peppers, seeded and finely chopped

1 tbsp garlic or herb vinegar
$\frac{1}{4}$ tsp grated lemon peel
2 tsp lemon juice
$\frac{1}{8}$ tsp cayenne pepper or chilli powder (optional)

Mix all ingredients thoroughly. Cover and refrigerate for 8 hours to blend flavours.

Total CHO = 20 g   Total Calories = 120

CRANBERRY RELISH

---

200 ml/7 fl oz unsweetened orange juice
350 g/12 oz fresh or frozen cranberries
2 tbsp grated orange peel

1 medium orange, peeled, sectioned and diced
1 medium apple, diced
non-nutritive intense sweetener to taste

Put orange juice into a large saucepan and heat to boiling. Add cranberries and boil, stirring occasionally, for 5 to 7 minutes. Remove from heat. Stir in orange peel, orange pieces and apple. Pour into a bowl and cool. Refrigerate for about 2 hours, sweetening to taste before serving.

Total CHO = 50 g   1 serving = 5 g CHO and 20
Total Calories = 200   calories
Serves 10

Children's Recipes

HAMBURGERS

450 g/1 lb lean minced beef
1 small onion, very finely
  chopped
½ tsp freshly ground pepper

½ tsp dry mustard
¼ tsp salt
4 tbsp iced water

Place all ingredients in a mixing bowl. Mix thoroughly with hands. Shape mixture into 4 patties, each about 8 cm/3 in across and 2.5 cm/1 in thick.

Heat grill to high. Place patties on grill rack and cook, about 10 cm/4 in from heat, for about 12 minutes or until done to taste, turning once.

Total CHO = negligible
Total Calories = 800
Serves 4

1 burger = negligible CHO
  and 200 calories

MOCK LASAGNE*

---

225 g/8 oz *wholemeal lasagne, broken into 2.5 cm/1 in pieces*
450 g/1 lb *lean minced beef*
2 tsp *salt*
¼ tsp *pepper*
¼ tsp *garlic salt*
400 g/14 oz *can chopped tomatoes, puréed*

1 tbsp *tomato purée*
225 g/8 oz *low-fat cottage cheese, sieved*
225 ml/8 fl oz *sour cream*
225 ml/8 fl oz *low-fat natural yogurt*
175 g/6 oz *Cheddar cheese, grated*

Cook lasagne as directed on packet. Heat oven to 180°C/350°F/mark 4.

Cook and stir minced beef, salt, pepper and garlic salt in a large frying pan until meat is brown. Drain off fat. Stir in tomatoes and tomato purée and simmer for 5 minutes. Stir in lasagne, cottage cheese, sour cream, yogurt and half the cheese. Pour into a casserole. Sprinkle remaining cheese on top. Bake for 35 to 40 minutes.

Total CHO = 200 g
Total Calories = 3120
Serves 8

1 serving = 25 g CHO and 390 calories

MEAT LOAF

---

450 g/1 lb *lean minced beef*
100 g/4 oz *ham, cut into 6 mm/¼ in cubes*
3 tbsp *chopped parsley*

1 egg, beaten
50 g/2 oz *porridge oats*
200 ml/7 fl oz *tomato juice*

Mix all ingredients thoroughly. Press mixture into a lightly oiled small loaf tin. Bake for 1 hour at 180°C/350°F/mark 4. Drain off any fat. Let stand for 5 minutes before turning out and slicing.

Total CHO = 40 g   1 serving = 5 g CHO and
Total Calories = 1200   150 calories
Serves 8

CHILLI CON CARNE*

450 g/1 lb lean minced beef   1 tbsp chilli powder
800 g/28 oz can whole   1 tsp salt
    tomatoes in tomato juice   1 tsp oregano
4 tbsp tomato purée   1 tsp Worcestershire sauce
2 medium onions, chopped   2 × 440 g/15½ oz cans red
1 clove garlic, crushed   kidney beans, drained

Cook and stir meat in a medium saucepan until brown. Drain any fat from pan. Add remaining ingredients, breaking up tomatoes with a fork.

Heat to boiling. Reduce heat, cover and simmer, stirring occasionally, for about 1½ hours.

Total CHO = 160 g   1 serving = 20 g CHO and
Total Calories = 1600   200 calories
Serves 8

BEAN SALAD*

Dressing (below)
440 g/15½ oz can chick peas, drained
440 g/15½ oz can red kidney beans, drained
440 g/15½ oz can white kidney beans (cannellini), drained

440 g/15½ oz can borlotti beans, drained
2 large onions, chopped
2 large carrots, peeled and diced
2–3 celery stalks, diced

Prepare dressing. Combine beans, onion, carrot and celery in a large bowl. Pour on dressing and mix. Cover and refrigerate for at least 4 hours to blend flavours.

Total CHO = 240 g
Total Calories = 2000
Serves 16

1 serving = 15 g CHO and 125 calories

Dressing

---

75 ml/⅛ pint olive oil
4 tbsp red wine vinegar
2 tsp dry mustard

pinch freshly ground pepper
1 tsp salt

Measure all ingredients into a screw-top jar. Cover and shake.

Total CHO = negligible   Total Calories = 680

SLOPPY JOES*

---

225 g/8 oz lean minced beef
1 small onion, chopped
½ small green pepper,
   seeded and chopped
2 medium tomatoes, skinned
   and chopped

275 ml/½ pint tomato juice
¼ tsp paprika
½ tsp salt
freshly ground pepper
4 wholemeal or granary
   baps

Cook and stir meat, onion and green pepper in large frying pan until meat is brown. Drain off any fat.

Stir in tomatoes, tomato juice, paprika and salt. Season with pepper. Heat to boiling. Reduce heat; cover and simmer for 15 to 20 minutes, stirring occasionally.

Cut baps horizontally into halves and toast. Top with meat mixture.

Total CHO = 100 g
Total Calories = 1000
Makes 4

Each 1 = 25 g CHO and 250
   calories

CHINESE PORK STEAKS*

---

1 egg
3 tbsp soy sauce
1 tbsp water or dry sherry
¼ tsp ginger
½ tsp garlic powder

75 g/3 oz fresh wholemeal
   bread, crumbed and dried
25 g/1 oz wheat germ
4 × 100 g/4 oz lean pork
   steaks, 2.5 cm/1 in thick

Beat egg, soy sauce, water, ginger and garlic powder in a shallow bowl or pie plate with a fork.

Mix breadcrumbs and wheat germ in another shallow dish.

Dip pork into egg mixture, then in breadcrumb mixture,

coating both sides. Place pork on lightly oiled Swiss roll tin.

Bake in a 180°C/350°F/mark 4 oven for 30 minutes. Turn pork carefully with a fish slice and bake for 20 minutes more or until tender.

Total CHO = 40 g
Total Calories = 1000
Serves 4

1 serving = 10 g CHO and
250 calories

EASY GRILLED CHICKEN

4 × 75 g/3 oz pieces boned
  chicken breast
2 tbsp finely chopped onion

4 tsp chopped parsley
4 tsp rosemary
salt and freshly ground
  pepper

Place each chicken piece on a 15 cm/6 in square of foil. Sprinkle each with the chopped onion, 1 tsp parsley, 1 tsp rosemary and a good pinch of pepper and salt. Fold foil over and seal each package securely.

Heat the grill to high. Cook the chicken, turning once, until tender; about 30 minutes.

Total CHO = negligible
Total Calories = 360
Serves 4

1 serving = negligible CHO
and 90 calories

FLAMBOYANT FISH

---

450 g/1 lb white fish fillets,
  thawed if frozen
1 tbsp grated onion
½ tsp salt
⅛ tsp pepper
1 medium tomato, skinned
  and chopped

1 medium green pepper,
  seeded and diced
25 g/1 oz margarine, melted
50 g/2 oz Emmental cheese,
  grated

Lightly oil a heat-proof serving dish. Arrange fillets on it in a single layer. Sprinkle with onion, salt and pepper. Cover fillets with tomato and green pepper; pour margarine over top.

Heat grill to high. Grill until fish flakes easily with a fork; 10 to 12 minutes. Remove from heat and sprinkle cheese on top. Return to grill for 2 to 3 minutes until cheese is melted.

Total CHO = negligible
Total Calories = 760
Serves 4

1 serving = negligible CHO
  and 190 calories

FISH IN FOIL

---

450 g/1 lb white fish fillets,
  thawed if frozen
350 g/12 oz carrots, peeled
  and thinly sliced
1 tbsp chopped onion

2 celery stalks, cut into 1
  cm/½ in pieces
1 lemon, cut into 8 slices
50 g/2 oz margarine
salt and freshly ground
  pepper

Heat oven to 200°C/400°F/mark 6. Cut fish into 4 pieces. Place in centre of a large sheet of foil laid on a baking sheet.

Cover fish with carrot, onion, celery and lemon slices. Dot with margarine. Season with salt and pepper. (If using fresh fish, sprinkle with 2 tbsp water.) Fold sides and ends of foil tightly around fish. Seal securely by pinching edges of foil together.

Bake until fish flakes easily with a fork; about 20 minutes.

Total CHO = 20 g   1 serving = 5 g CHO and
Total Calories = 800   200 calories
Serves 4

HAM AND MACARONI BAKE*

225 g/8 oz wholemeal macaroni
50 g/2 oz margarine
25 g/1 oz plain flour
2 tbsp mustard
¼ tsp salt
pinch pepper
425 ml/¾ pint skimmed milk

225 g/8 oz cooked lean ham, cubed
2 medium apples, peeled, cored and thinly sliced
75 g/3 oz fresh wholemeal bread, crumbed
25 g/1 oz margarine, melted

Cook macaroni as directed on packet.

Melt margarine in a large saucepan. Stir in flour, mustard, salt and pepper. Cook over a low heat, stirring, until mixture is smooth and bubbly. Remove from heat. Stir in milk. Heat to boiling, stirring constantly. Boil and stir for 1 minute. Stir in macaroni, ham and apple; pour into a large casserole.

Mix breadcrumbs and the melted margarine; sprinkle on the casserole. Bake in a 180°C/350°F/mark 4 oven for 30 to 35 minutes, until hot and bubbly.

Total CHO = 240 g
Total Calories = 2000
Serves 8

1 serving = 30 g CHO and
250 calories

STRAWBERRY MILK SMOOTHEE

275 ml/½ pint skimmed
  milk
225 g/8 oz strawberries,
  sliced

1 tsp vanilla essence
1 tsp lemon juice
nutmeg (optional)

Measure all ingredients into a blender. Cover and process at high speed until smooth. Pour into glasses and, if desired, sprinkle with ground nutmeg.

Total CHO = 30 g
Total Calories = 150
Serves 2

1 serving = 15 g CHO and
75 calories

BLENDER BANANA

275 ml/½ pint skimmed
  milk
1 tsp vanilla essence

150 g/5 oz banana, peeled
  and chopped

Place all ingredients in blender. Cover and process at high speed until smooth; about 10 seconds. Pour into 2 glasses or dessert dishes. Serve immediately or freeze for dessert.

Total CHO = 30 g
Total Calories = 160
Serves 2

1 serving = 15 g CHO and
80 calories

EVER-READY SNACK

---

225 g/8 oz sultanas
225 g/8 oz raisins
100 g/4 oz currants

100 g/4 oz sunflower seeds
225 g/8 oz dry-roasted
  peanuts

Mix all ingredients in a large bowl. Store in an air-tight container.

Total CHO = 400 g
Total Calories = 3200
Serves 8

1 serving = 50 g CHO and
  400 calories

ANDREW'S DELUXE PEANUT BUTTER

---

150 g/5 oz carrot, peeled and
  coarsely grated
200 g/7 oz crunchy peanut
  butter
2 tbsp reduced-calorie
  mayonnaise

50 g/2 oz hulled sunflower
  seeds
75 g/3 oz raisins

Measure all ingredients into a bowl. Mix thoroughly. Store in a covered container in the refrigerator.

Total CHO = 100 g

Total Calories = 1800

TUNA SALAD SANDWICHES

---

200 g/7 oz can tuna in brine,
drained
2 tbsp finely chopped celery
1 tbsp very finely chopped
onion

4 tbsp reduced-calorie
mayonnaise
freshly ground pepper
6 small thin slices
wholemeal bread

Empty tuna into a bowl and flake with a fork. Add celery, onion and mayonnaise and season with a dash of pepper. Mix lightly with a fork until ingredients are coated.

Divide mixture between 3 slices of bread. Top each with another slice. Press together and cut in half.

Total CHO = 60 g
Total Calories = 660
Makes 3 sandwiches

1 sandwich = 20 g CHO and
220 calories

FROZEN FRUIT CUPS

---

1 large orange, peeled,
sectioned and cut up
150 g/5 oz strawberries

425 ml/¾ pint unsweetened
orange juice

Divide orange pieces and strawberries among 6 small plastic cups. Pour orange juice over fruit. Place in freezer until partially frozen.

Insert a lolly stick in each cup and return to freezer.

Remove ice from cups by pushing up on bottom of cup until it slides out.

Total CHO = 60 g
Total Calories = 270
Serves 6

1 serving = 10 g CHO and
45 calories

SUMMER FROZEN FRUIT

---

3 peaches, peeled and sliced
225 g/8 oz strawberries,
   halved

225 g/8 oz raspberries
700 ml/1¼ pints
   unsweetened orange juice

Arrange fruits in a small baking tin. Pour in orange juice. Cover with foil and freeze. To serve, cut into 6 squares.

Total CHO = 120 g
Total Calories = 510
Serves 6

1 serving = 20 g CHO and
   85 calories

NUTTY ORANGE OATMEAL BISCUITS

---

75 g/3 oz margarine,
   softened
150 g/5.3 oz pot low-fat
   natural yogurt
50 g/2 oz brown sugar
1 tsp vanilla essence
150 g/5 oz wholemeal flour

75 g/3 oz porridge oats
¼ tsp bicarbonate of soda
25 g/1 oz walnuts, finely
   chopped
¼ tsp grated orange peel

Heat oven to 170°C/325°F/mark 3. Blend margarine, yogurt, sugar and vanilla essence. Mix in remaining ingredients. Shape dough by rounded teaspoonfuls into 2.5 cm/1 in balls (makes about 50). Place about 5 cm/2 in apart on an ungreased baking sheet; flatten slightly with a fork.

Bake for 12 to 15 minutes until pale golden brown. Remove from baking sheet immediately.

Nutty Orange Oatmeal Balls: Place balls 2.5 cm/1 in apart on baking sheet. Do not flatten. Bake as above.

Total CHO = 250 g
Total Calories = 1750
Makes about 50 biscuits

1 biscuit = 5 g CHO and 35
calories

NEW-FASHION OATMEAL BISCUITS

100 g/4 oz plain flour
50 g/2 oz wholemeal flour
75 g/3 oz porridge oats
1 tsp baking powder
½ tsp salt
¼ tsp bicarbonate of soda
⅛ tsp ginger
½ tsp grated orange or
lemon peel
75 g/3 oz coarsely chopped
nuts

2 tbsp sesame seed
100 g/4 oz raisins
450 g/1 lb ripe peeled
bananas
75 g/3 oz margarine,
softened
1 egg
25 g/1 oz dried non-fat
skimmed milk

Heat oven to 200°C/400°F/mark 6. Lightly oil a baking sheet.

Measure flours, oats, baking powder, salt, bicarbonate of soda, ginger, orange peel, nuts, sesame seed and raisins into a bowl and set aside.

Mash bananas by slicing them into a large mixer bowl and beat at low speed, scraping bowl constantly. Increase speed to medium and beat until mixture is smooth. Add remaining ingredients; beat until smooth, scraping bowl occasionally.

Remove beater. Mix in flour mixture with a spoon. Drop dough by teaspoonfuls on to baking sheet (48 biscuits in all).

Bake for about 10 minutes or until golden brown. Cool on a wire rack.

Total CHO = 360 g
Total Calories = 2640
Makes 48

1 serving of 2 biscuits = 15 g
CHO and 110 calories

Index of
Medical References

Index of Recipes